J.-P. Lepoittevin

C. J. Le Coz

Dictionary of C

J.-P. Lepoittevin
C. J. Le Coz

Dictionary of Contact Allergens

With a Contribution by Peter J. Frosch

With 4 Figures in Color and 12 Tables

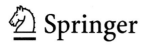 Springer

Lepoittevin, Jean-Pierre, Professor
(e-mail: jplepoit@chimie.u-strasbg.fr)
Laboratoire de Dermato-Chimie
Clinique Dermatologique, CHU
67091 Strasbourg Cedex, France

Le Coz, Christophe J.
(e-mail: christophe.lecoz@wanadoo.fr)
Unité Dermato-Allergologie
Hôpitaux Universitaires de Strasbourg
1, Place de l'Hôpital
67091 Strasbourg
France

This book is based on Frosch, Menné, Lepoittevin "Contact Dermatitis, 4th Edition", ISBN 978-3-540-24471-4

Library of Congress Control Number: 2007932601

ISBN 978-3-540-74164-0 Springer Berlin Heidelberg New York

Springer is a part of Springer Science+Business Media
springer.com
© Springer-Verlag Berlin Heidelberg 2007
Printed in Germany

Editor: Marion Philipp, Heidelberg, Germany
Desk Editor: Ellen Blasig, Heidelberg, Germany
Cover: Frido-Steinen-Broo, EStudio, Calamar, Spain
Typesetting: K. Detzner, 67346 Speyer, Germany
Production: LE-TeX Jelonek, Schmidt & Vöckler GbR, Leipzig, Germany

Printed on acid-free paper   24/3180/YL   5 4 3 2 1 0

Preface

Chemistry plays a major role in our understanding of allergic contact dermatitis (ACD), but playing with molecules is not always an easy task for nonspecialists. This book has been written to familiarize the reader with the structures of some of the chemicals involved in ACD. We have attempted to provide useful information for those who would like to find out more from the literature or on the internet: the principal name; the most important synonym(s); the Chemical Abstract Service (CAS) registry number, which is the identity number of a molecule; and a few relevant literature references. Considering the chemical structure of one molecule and comparing it with that of another is the only way to discuss possible cross-reactions when several patch tests are positive in the same patient.

Most of the molecules listed in this book are not in the European Standard series, nor are they in the more specialized batteries, but experience shows that patients can be exposed to them in their environment. Therefore, we have added to this dictionary of contact allergens some guidelines on patch testing with the patients' own products.

Welcome to the world of chemistry!

Strasbourg, August 2007
Jean-Pierre Lepoittevin
Christophe J. Le Coz

Contents

Dictionary of Contact Allergens: Chemical Structures, Sources and References

Christophe J. Le Coz, Jean-Pierre Lepoittevin

1.1 Introduction

This chapter has been written in order to familiarize the reader with the chemical structure of chemicals implicated in contact dermatitis, mainly as haptens responsible for allergic contact dermatitis. For each molecule, the principal name is used for classification. We have also listed the most important synonym(s), the Chemical Abstract Service (CAS) Registry Number that characterizes the substance, and its chemical structure. The reader will find one or more relevant literature references. As it was not possible to be exhaustive, some allergens have been omitted since they were obsolete, extremely rarely implicated in contact dermatitis, their case reports were too imprecise, or they are extensively treated in other chapters of the textbook. From a practical chemical point of view, acrylates, cyanoacrylates and (meth)acrylates, cephalosporins, and parabens have been grouped together.

1. Abietic acid

CAS Registry Number [514–10–3]

Abietic acid is probably the major allergen of colophony, along with dehydroabietic acid, by way of oxidation products. Its detection in a material indicates that allergenic components of colophony are present.

Suggested Reading

Bergh M, Menné T, Karlberg AT (1994) Colophony in paper-based surgical clothing. Contact Dermatitis 31:332–333

Karlberg AT, Bergstedt E, Boman A, Bohlinder K, Lidén C, Nilsson JLG, Wahlberg JE (1985) Is abietic acid the allergenic component of colophony? Contact Dermatitis 13:209–215

Karlberg AT, Bohlinder K, Boman A, Hacksell U, Hermansson J, Jacobsson S, Nilsson JLG (1988) Identification of 15-hydroperoxyabietic acid as a contact allergen in Portuguese colophony. J Pharm Pharmacol 40: 42–47

2. Acetaldehyde

Acetic Aldehyde, Ethanal, Ethylic Aldehyde

CAS Registry Number [75–07–0]

Acetaldehyde, as its metabolite, is responsible for many of the effects of ethanol, such as hepatic or neurological toxicity. A case of contact allergy was reported in the textile industry, where dimethoxane was used as a biocide agent in textiles and its degradation led to acetaldehyde.

Suggested Reading

Eriksson CJ (2001) The role of acetaldehyde in the actions of alcohol (update 2000). Alcohol Clin Exp Res 25 [Suppl 5]:15S–32S

Shmunes E, Kempton RJ (1980) Allergic contact dermatitis to dimethoxane in a spin finish. Contact Dermatitis 6:421–424

3. Acrylamide

CAS Registry Number [79–06–1]

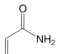

Acrylamide is used in the plastic polymers industry, for water treatments, soil stabilization, and to prepare polyacrylamide gels for electrophoresis. This neurotoxic, carcinogenic, and genotoxic substance is known to have caused contact dermatitis in industrial and laboratory workers.

Suggested Reading

Beyer DJ, Belsito DV (2000) Allergic contact dermatitis from acrylamide in a chemical mixer. Contact Dermatitis 42:181–182

Dooms-Goossens A, Garmyn M, Degreef H (1991) Contact allergy to acrylamide. Contact Dermatitis 24:71–72

Lambert J, Mathieu L, Dockx P (1988) Contact dermatitis from acrylamide. Contact Dermatitis 19:65

4. Acrylates, Cyanoacrylate, and Methacrylates

Acrylic Acid and Acrylates

CAS Registry Number
[79–10–7]

Acrylic acid

Acrylate

Acrylates are esters from acrylic acid. Occupational contact allergies from acrylates have frequently been reported and mainly concern workers exposed to the glues based on acrylic acid, as well as dental workers and beauticians.

Bisphenol A Diglycidylether Diacrylate

2,2-bis[4-(2-Hydroxy-3-Acryloxypropoxy)phenyl]-Propane (Bis-GA)

CAS Registry Number [8687–94–9]

Bis-GA is an epoxy diacrylate. It caused contact dermatitis in a process worker, being contained in ultraviolet-light-curable acrylic paints.

Suggested Reading
Jolanki R, Kanerva L, Estlander T (1995) Occupational allergic contact
dermatitis caused by epoxy diacrylate in ultraviolet-light-cured paint,
and bisphenol A in dental composite resin. Contact Dermatitis 33:
94–99

Bisphenol A Glycidyl Methacrylate

Bis-GMA

CAS Registry Number [1565–94–2]

Bis-GMA is an epoxy-methacrylate. Sensitization occurs in dentists, in beauticians, and in consumers with sculptured photopolymerizable nails.

Suggested Reading
Kanerva L, Estlander T, Jolanki R (1989) Allergic contact dermatitis from
dental composite resins due to aromatic epoxy acrylates and aliphatic
acrylates. Contact Dermatitis 20:201–211

1,4-Butanediol Diacrylate

CAS Registry Number [1070–70–8]

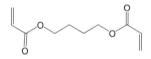

A positive patch test was observed in a male process worker in a
paint factory, sensitized to an epoxy diacrylate contained in raw
materials of ultraviolet-light-curable paint. The positive reaction
was probably due to a cross-reactivity.

Suggested Reading
Jolanki R, Kanerva L, Estlander T (1995) Occupational allergic contact
dermatitis caused by epoxy diacrylate in ultraviolet-light-cured paint,
and bisphenol A in dental composite resin. Contact Dermatitis 33:
94–99

1,4-Butanediol Dimethacrylate

CAS Registry Number
[141–32–2]

Sensitization to 1,4-butanediol dimethacrylate was reported in dental technicians, with cross-reactivity to methyl methacrylate.

Suggested Reading
Rustemeyer T, Frosch PJ (1996) Occupational skin diseases in dental laboratory technicians. (I). Clinical picture and causative factors. Contact Dermatitis 34:125–133

n-Butyl Acrylate

CAS Registry Number
[141–32–2]

Sensitization to *n*-butyl acrylate can occur in the dental profession.

Suggested Reading
Daecke C, Schaller J, Goos M (1994) Acrylates as potent allergens in occupational and domestic exposures. Contact Dermatitis 30:190–191
Kanerva L, Estlander T, Jolanki R, Tarvainen K (1993) Occupational allergic contact dermatitis caused by exposure to acrylates during work with dental prostheses. Contact Dermatitis 28:268–275
Rustemeyer T, Frosch PJ (1996) Occupational skin diseases in dental laboratory technicians. (I). Clinical picture and causative factors. Contact Dermatitis 34:125–133

tert-Butyl Acrylate

CAS Registry Number
[1663–39–4]

Sensitization may affect dental workers.

Suggested Reading
Kanerva L, Estlander T, Jolanki R, Tarvainen K (1993) Occupational allergic contact dermatitis caused by exposure to acrylates during work with dental prostheses. Contact Dermatitis 28:268–275

Cyanoacrylic Acid and Cyanoacrylates

2-Cyanoacrylic Acid

CAS Registry Number [15802–18–3]

Cyanoacrylic acid   Cyanoacrylate

Cyanoacrylates, particularly 2-ethyl cyanoacrylate, are derived from cyanoacrylic acid. They are used as sealants.

Suggested Reading
Fischer AA (1985) Reactions to cyanoacrylate adhesives: "instant glue".
 Cutis 35:18, 20, 22
Tarvainen K (1995) Analysis of patients with allergic patch test reactions
 to a plastics and glue series. Contact Dermatitis 32:346–351

Diethyleneglycol Diacrylate

CAS Registry Number [4074–88–8]

Diethyleneglycol diacrylate was positive in a painter sensitized to his own acrylate-based paint.

Suggested Reading
Nakamura M, Arima Y, Yoneda K, Nobuhara S, Miyachi Y (1999) Occupa-
 tional contact dermatitis from acrylic monomer in paint. Contact
 Dermatitis 40:228–229

Ethyl Acrylate

CAS Registry Number [140–88–5]

Ethyl acrylate is a sensitizer in the dental profession.

Suggested Reading

Kanerva L, Estlander T, Jolanki R, Tarvainen K (1993) Occupational allergic contact dermatitis caused by exposure to acrylates during work with dental prostheses. Contact Dermatitis 28:268–275

Rustemeyer T, Frosch PJ (1996) Occupational skin diseases in dental laboratory technicians. (I). Clinical picture and causative factors. Contact Dermatitis 34:125–133

Ethyl Cyanoacrylate

Ethyl-2-Cyanoacrylate

CAS Registry Number [7085–85–0]

Ethyl cyanoacrylate is contained in instant glues for metal, glass, rubber, plastics, textiles, tissues, and nails. It polymerizes almost instantaneously in air at room temperature and bonds immediately and strongly to surface keratin. Beauticians are exposed to contact dermatitis from nail glues.

Suggested Reading

Bruze M, Björkner B, Lepoittevin JP (1995) Occupational allergic contact dermatitis from ethyl cyanoacrylate. Contact Dermatitis 32:156–159

Fitzgerald DA, Bhaggoe R, English JSC (1995) Contact sensitivity to cyanoacrylate nail-adhesive with dermatitis at remote sites. Contact Dermatitis 32:175–176

Jacobs MC, Rycroft RJG (1995) Allergic contact dermatitis from cyanoacrylate? Contact Dermatitis 33:71

Tomb R, Lepoittevin JP, Durepaire F, Grosshans E (1993) Ectopic contact dermatitis from ethyl cyanoacrylate instant adhesives. Contact Dermatitis 28:206–208

Ethyleneglycol Dimethacrylate

CAS Registry Number [97–90–5]

Ethyleneglycol dimethacrylate (EGDMA) is a cross-linking agent of acrylic resins and is employed to optimize the dilution of high-viscosity monomers and to link together the macromolecules constituting the polymer. It caused contact dermatitis in dental technicians and dental assistants. A case was also reported in a manufacturer of car rearview mirrors.

Suggested Reading

Farli M, Gasperini M, Francalanci S, Gola M, Sertoli A (1990) Occupational contact dermatitis in 2 dental technicians. Contact Dermatitis 22: 282–287

Kanerva L, Jolanki R, Estlander T (1995) Occupational allergic contact dermatitis from 2-hydroxyethyl methacrylate and ethylene glycol dimethacrylate in a modified acrylic structural adhesive. Contact Dermatitis 35:84–89

Rustemeyer T, Frosch PJ (1996) Occupational skin diseases in dental laboratory technicians. (I). Clinical picture and causative factors. Contact Dermatitis 34:125–133

Tosti A, Rapacchiale S, Piraccini BM, Peluso AM (1991) Occupational airborne contact dermatitis due to ethylene glycol dimethacrylate. Contact Dermatitis 24:152–153

2-Ethylhexyl Acrylate

2-EHA

CAS Registry Number [1322–13–0]

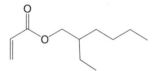

2-EHA was contained in a surgical tape and caused allergic contact dermatitis in a patient.

Suggested Reading

Daecke C, Schaller J, Goos M (1994) Acrylates as potent allergens in occupational and domestic exposures. Contact Dermatitis 30:190–191

Ethyl Methacrylate

CAS Registry Number [97–63–2].

Ethyl methacrylate is used in dental prostheses or in photobonded sculptured nails.

Suggested Reading

Kanerva L, Estlander T, Jolanki R, Tarvainen K (1993) Occupational allergic contact dermatitis caused by exposure to acrylates during work with dental prostheses. Contact Dermatitis 28:268–275

Kanerva L, Lauerma A, Estlander T, Alanko K, Henriks-Eckerman ML, Jolanki R (1996) Occupational allergic contact dermatitis caused by photobonded sculptured nails and a review of (meth) acrylates in nail cosmetics. Am J Contact Dermat 7:109–115

Rustemeyer T, Frosch PJ (1996) Occupational skin diseases in dental laboratory technicians. (I). Clinical picture and causative factors. Contact Dermatitis 34:125–133

Glycidyl Methacrylate

CAS Registry Number [106–91–2]

Glycidyl methacrylate was reported as the allergenic component of the anaerobic sealant Sta-Lok.

Suggested Reading

Dempsey KJ (1982) Hypersensitivity to Sta-Lok and Loctite anaerobic sealants. J Am Acad Dermatol 7:779–784

1,6-Hexanediol Diacrylate
Hexamethylene Diacrylate

CAS Registry Number [13048–33–4]

Sensitization occurred after accidental occupational exposure in an employee in the laboratory of a plastic paint factory.

Suggested Reading

Botella-Estrada R, Mora E, de La Cuadra J (1992) Hexanediol diacrylate sensitization after accidental occupational exposure. Contact Dermatitis 26:50–51

2-Hydroxyethyl Acrylate
2-HEA, Ethylene Glycol Acrylate

CAS Registry Number [818–61–1]

2-HEA is contained in Lowicryl 4KM and K11 M resins. It caused contact dermatitis in workers embedding media for electron microscopy. It may also be contained in UV-cured nail gel used for photobonded, sculptured nails.

Suggested Reading

Kanerva L, Lauerma A, Estlander T, Alanko K, Henriks-Eckerman ML, Jolanki R (1996) Occupational allergic contact dermatitis caused by photobonded sculptured nails and a review of (meth) acrylates in nail cosmetics. Am J Contact Dermat 7:109–115

Tobler M, Wüthrich B, Freiburghaus AU (1990) Contact dermatitis from acrylate and methacrylate compounds in Lowicryl® embedding media for electron microscopy. Contact Dermatitis 23:96–102

2-Hydroxyethyl Methacrylate

2-HEMA

CAS Registry Number [868–77–9]

Sensitization to 2-HEMA concerns mainly dental technicians and dentists, but can also occur in other workers such as printers or beauticians or consumers using photopolymerizable sculptured nails.

Suggested Reading

Geukens S, Goossens A (2001) Occupational contact allergy to (meth)-acrylates. Contact Dermatitis 44:153–159

Jolanki R, Kanerva L, Estlander T, Tarvainen K (1994) Concomitant sensitization to triglycidyl isocyanurate, diaminodiphenylmethane and 2-hydroxyethyl methacrylate from silk-screen printing coatings in the manufacture of circuit boards. Contact Dermatitis 30:12–15

Kanerva L, Estlander T, Jolanki R, Tarvainen K (1993) Occupational allergic contact dermatitis caused by exposure to acrylates during work with dental prostheses. Contact Dermatitis 28:268–275

Kanerva L, Jolanki R, Estlander T (1995) Occupational allergic contact dermatitis from 2-hydroxyethyl methacrylate and ethylene glycol dimethacrylate in a modified acrylic structural adhesive. Contact Dermatitis 35:84–89

Rustemeyer T, Frosch PJ (1996) Occupational skin diseases in dental laboratory technicians. (I). Clinical picture and causative factors. Contact Dermatitis 34:125–133

2-Hydroxypropyl Acrylate

CAS Registry Number
[999–61–1]

A case of occupational contact dermatitis was reported in industry.

Suggested Reading
Lovell CR, Rycroft RJG, Williams DMJ, Hamlin JW (1985) Contact derma-
    titis from the irritancy (immediate and delayed) and allergenicity of
    hydroxypropyl acrylate. Contact Dermatitis 12 : 117–118

2-Hydroxypropyl Methacrylate

CAS Registry Number [27813–02–1]

Sensitization to 2-hydroxypropyl methacrylate concerns mainly
the dental profession.

Suggested Reading
Kanerva L, Estlander T, Jolanki R, Tarvainen K (1993) Occupational aller-
    gic contact dermatitis caused by exposure to acrylates during work
    with dental prostheses. Contact Dermatitis 28 : 268–275
Kanerva L, Estlander T, Jolanki R (1997) Occupational allergic contact
    dermatitis caused by triacrylic tri-cure glass ionomer. Contact Derma-
    titis 37 : 49
Rustemeyer T, Frosch PJ (1996) Occupational skin diseases in dental lab-
    oratory technicians. (I). Clinical picture and causative factors. Contact
    Dermatitis 34 : 125–133

Methacrylic Acid and Methacrylates

CAS Registry Number [79–41–4]

Methacrylic acid   Methacrylate

Methacrylates are derived from methacrylic acid. They are used in
the production of a great variety of polymers. As they are moderate to strong sensitizers, sensitization concerns many professions.
Dental technicians, assistants, and surgeons are frequently exposed. Methacrylates were reported as occupational allergens in
chemically cured or photocured sculptured nails.

Methyl Acrylate

MA

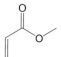

CAS Registry Number [96–33–3].

MA is contained in some nail lacquers.

Suggested Reading

Kanerva L, Estlander T, Jolanki R, Tarvainen K (1993) Occupational allergic contact dermatitis caused by exposure to acrylates during work with dental prostheses. Contact Dermatitis 28:268–275

Kanerva L, Lauerma A, Estlander T, Alanko K, Henriks-Eckerman ML, Jolanki R (1996) Occupational allergic contact dermatitis caused by photobonded sculptured nails and a review of (meth) acrylates in nail cosmetics. Am J Contact Dermat 7:109–115

Methyl Methacrylate and Polymethyl Methacrylate

CAS Registry Numbers [80–62–6] and [9011–14–7]

Methyl methacrylate is one of the most common methacrylates. This acrylic monomer, the essential component of the fluid mixed with the powder, causes allergic contact dermatitis mainly in dental technicians and dentists. Cases were also reported following the use of sculptured nails and in ceramic workers. Polymethyl methacrylate is the result of polymerized methyl methacrylate monomers, which are used as sheets, molding, extrusion powders, surface coating resins, emulsion polymers, fibers, inks, and films. This material is also used in tooth implants, bone cements, and hard corneal contact lenses.

Suggested Reading

Farli M, Gasperini M, Francalanci S, Gola M, Sertoli A (1990) Occupational contact dermatitis in 2 dental technicians. Contact Dermatitis 22:282–287

Gebhardt M, Geier J (1996) Evaluation of patch test results with denture material series. Contact Dermatitis 34:191–195

Kanerva L, Estlander T, Jolanki R, Tarvainen K (1993) Occupational allergic contact dermatitis caused by exposure to acrylates during work with dental prostheses. Contact Dermatitis 28:268–275

Kanerva L, Lauerma A, Estlander T, Alanko K, Henriks-Eckerman ML, Jolanki R (1996) Occupational allergic contact dermatitis caused by photobonded sculptured nails and a review of (meth) acrylates in nail cosmetics. Am J Contact Dermat 7:109–115

Kiec-Swierczynska MK (1996) Occupational allergic contact dermatitis due to acrylates in Lodz. Contact Dermatitis 34:419–422

Rustemeyer T, Frosch PJ. Occupational skin diseases in dental laboratory technicians. (I). Clinical picture and causative factors. Contact Dermatitis. 34:125–133

Pentaerythrityl Triacrylate

CAS Registry Numbers [3524–68–3] and others

Pentaerythritol triacrylate is a multifunctional acrylic monomer. It can be contained in photopolymerizable printer's ink or varnishes. Sensitization was described in dental technicians and in a textile fabric printer.

Suggested Reading

Geukens S, Goossens A (2001) Occupational contact allergy to (meth)-acrylates. Contact Dermatitis 44:153–159

Kanerva L, Estlander T, Jolanki R, Tarvainen K (1995) Occupational allergic contact dermatitis and contact urticaria caused by polyfunctional aziridine hardener. Contact Dermatitis 33:304–309

Kiec-Swierczynska MK (1996) Occupational allergic contact dermatitis due to acrylates in Lodz. Contact Dermatitis 34:419–422

Rustemeyer T, Frosch PJ (1996) Occupational skin diseases in dental laboratory technicians. (I). Clinical picture and causative factors. Contact Dermatitis 34:125–133

Polyurethane Dimethacrylate

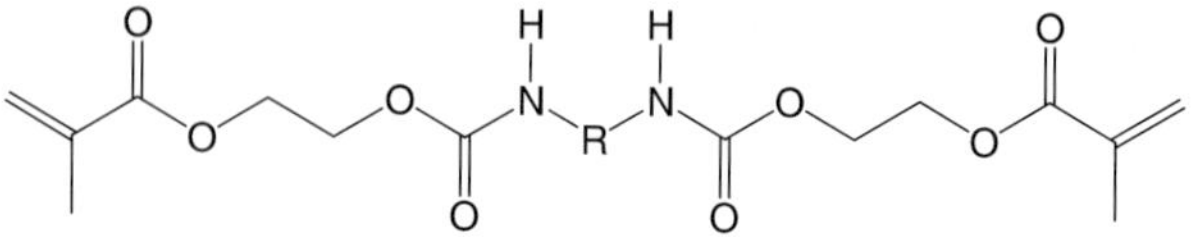

R =   or

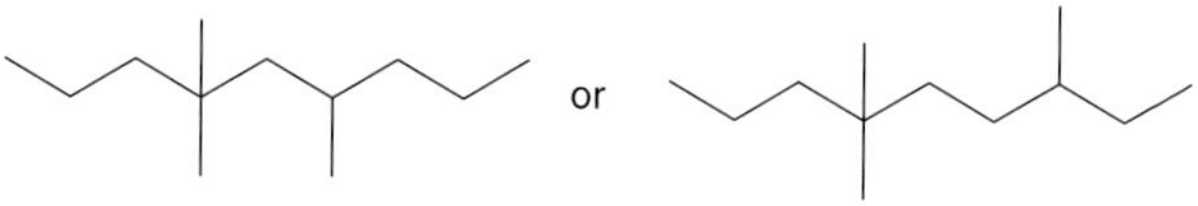

The polyurethane dimethacrylate was contained in Loctite glues of the 300 and 500 series.

Suggested Reading
Dempsey KJ (1982) Hypersensitivity to Sta-Lok and Loctite anaerobic sealants. J Am Acad Dermatol 7:779–784

Tetraethylene Glycol Dimethacrylate

CAS Registry Number [109–17–1]

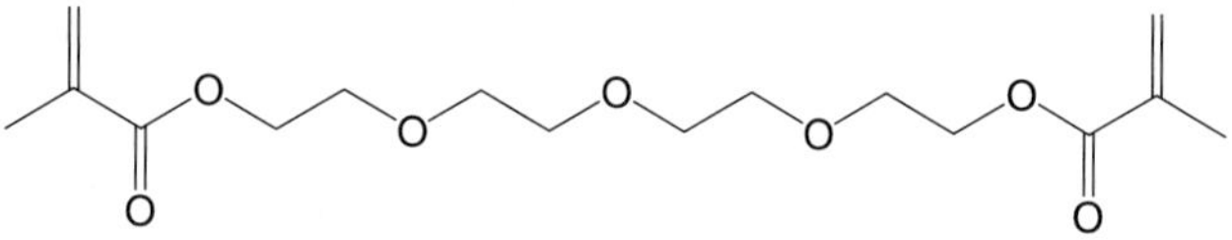

Tetraethylene glycol dimethacrylate is a crosslinking agent of acrylic resins, employed to optimize the dilution of high-viscosity monomers and to link together the macromolecules constituting the polymer, to make the three-dimensional structure more rigid. Occupational dermatitis was reported in a dental technician.

Suggested Reading
Farli M, Gasperini M, Francalanci S, Gola M, Sertoli A (1990) Occupational contact dermatitis in 2 dental technicians. Contact Dermatitis 22: 282–287

Triethylene Glycol Dimethacrylate

CAS Registry Number [109–16–0]

Triethylene glycol dimethacrylate (TREGDMA) is a cross-linking agent of acrylic resins, used in sealants or in dental bonding resins. It is mainly used in dentistry, by dental technicians and dentists.

Suggested Reading

Farli M, Gasperini M, Francalanci S, Gola M, Sertoli A (1990) Occupational contact dermatitis in 2 dental technicians. Contact Dermatitis 22: 282–287

Kanerva L, Lauerma A, Estlander T, Alanko K, Henriks-Eckerman ML, Jolanki R (1996) Occupational allergic contact dermatitis caused by photobonded sculptured nails and a review of (meth) acrylates in nail cosmetics. Am J Contact Dermat 7:109–115

Kiec-Swierczynska MK (1996) Occupational allergic contact dermatitis due to acrylates in Lodz. Contact Dermatitis 34:419–422

Rustemeyer T, Frosch PJ (1996) Occupational skin diseases in dental laboratory technicians. (I). Clinical picture and causative factors. Contact Dermatitis 34:125–133

Trimethylolpropane Triacrylate

CAS Registry Number [15625–89–5]

Trimethylolpropane triacrylate (TMPTA) is a multifunctional acrylic monomer. It reacts with propyleneimine to form polyfunctional aziridine. Sensitization was observed in a textile fabric printer. Patch tests were positive with the polyfunctional aziridine hardener, but were negative to TMPTA. TMPTA caused contact dermatitis in an optic fibre manufacturing worker and was reported as a sensitizer in a floor top coat or in photopolymerizable inks.

Suggested Reading

Kanerva L, Estlander T, Jolanki R, Tarvainen K (1995) Occupational aller-
    gic contact dermatitis and contact urticaria caused by polyfunctional
    aziridine hardener. Contact Dermatitis 33:304–309
Kiec-Swierczynska MK (1996) Occupational allergic contact dermatitis
    due to acrylates in Lodz. Contact Dermatitis 34:419–422
Maurice PDL, Rycroft RJG (1986) Allergic contact dermatitis from UV
    curing acrylate in the manufacture of optical fibres. Contact Derma-
    titis 15:92–93

Tripropylene Glycol Diacrylate

CAS Registry Number [42978–66–5]

As a cause of occupational contact dermatitis, tripropylene glycol
diacrylate was contained in dental resins, in UV-cured inks and in
nail cosmetics.

Suggested Reading

Kanerva L, Estlander T, Jolanki R, Tarvainen K (1993) Occupational aller-
    gic contact dermatitis caused by exposure to acrylates during work
    with dental prostheses. Contact Dermatitis 28:268–275
Kanerva L, Lauerma A, Estlander T, Alanko K, Henriks-Eckerman ML,
    Jolanki R (1996) Occupational allergic contact dermatitis caused by
    photobonded sculptured nails and a review of (meth)acrylates in nail
    cosmetics. Am J Contact Dermat 7:109–115

Urethane Acrylate

R =

Urethane acrylate gave a positive reaction in a lottery-ticket-coating machine worker sensitized to epoxy acrylate oligomers contained in a UV varnish.

Suggested Reading

Guimaraens D, Gonzalez MA, del Rio E, Condé-Salazar L (1994) Occupational airborne allergic contact dermatitis in the national mint and fiscal-stamp factory. Contact Dermatitis 30:172–173

Kanerva L, Estlander T, Jolanki R, Tarvainen K (1993) Occupational allergic contact dermatitis caused by exposure to acrylates during work with dental prostheses. Contact Dermatitis 28:268–275

5. Acrylonitrile

2-Propenenitrile

CAS Registry Number [107–13–1]

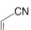

Acrylonitrile is a raw material used extensively in industry, mainly for acrylic and modacrylic fibres, acrylonitrile-butadiene-styrene and styrene-acrylonitrile resins, adiponitrile used in nylon's synthesis, for nitrile rubber, and plastics. It is also used as an insecticide. This very toxic and irritant substance is also a sensitizer and caused both irritant and allergic contact dermatitis in a production manufacturer.

Suggested Reading

Bakker JG, Jongen SMJ, Van Neer FCJ, Neis JM (1991) Occupational contact dermatitis due to acrylonitrile. Contact Dermatitis 24:50–53

Chu CY, Sun CC (2001) Allergic contact dermatitis from acrylonitrile. Am J Contact Dermat 12:113–114

6. Alachlor®

2-Chloro-2′,6′-Diethyl-N-(Methoxymethyl)-Acetanilide, 2-Chloro-N-(2,6-Diethylphenyl)-N-(Methoxymethyl)Acetamide

CAS Registry Number [15972–60–8]

Alachlor® is a herbicide. Occupational contact dermatitis was rarely observed in agricultural workers.

Suggested Reading
Won JH, Ahn SK, Kim SC (1993) Allergic contact dermatitis from the herbicide Alachlor®. Contact Dermatitis 28:38–39

7. Alantolactone

CAS Registry Number [546–43–0]

The allergen eudesmanolide sesquiterpene lactone was isolated from elecampane (*Inula helenium* L.). With dehydrocostuslactone and costunolide, it is a component of the (sesquiterpene) lactone mix used to detect sensitization to Compositae–Asteraceae.

Suggested Reading
Ducombs G, Benezra C, Talaga P, Andersen KE, Burrows D, Camarasa JG, Dooms-Goossens A, Frosch PJ, Lachapelle JM, Menné T, Rycroft RJG, White IR, Shaw S, Wilkinson JD (1990) Patch testing with the "sesquiterpene lactone mix": a marker for contact allergy to Compositae and other sesquiterpene-lactone-containing plants. Contact Dermatitis 22: 249–252
Lamminpää A, Estlander T, Jolanki R, Kanerva L (1996) Occupational allergic contact dermatitis caused by decorative plants. Contact Dermatitis 34:330–335

8. Alkyl Glucosides

Alkyl glucosides are copolymers; based on a fatty alcohol and a glucoside polymer, they comprise decyl glucoside, coco glucoside and lauryl (dodecyl) glucoside in cosmetics, and cetearyl glucoside as a surfactant and emulsifying agent because of its higher viscosity. Due to their manufacturing processes, they are blends of several copolymers. For example, coco glucoside contains C_6, C_8, C_{10}, C_{12}, C_{14}, and C_{16} fatty alcohols. Such variations explain uncertainty when searching for the precise CAS Registry Number. Because alkyl glucosides are comparable mixtures, patients sensitive to one alkyl glucoside may also react to others. See also 127. Decyl Glucoside.

Suggested Reading
Goossens A, Decraene T, Platteaux N, Nardelli A, Rasschaert V (2003) Glucosides as unexpected allergens in cosmetics. Contact Dermatitis 48:164–166
Le Coz CJ, Meyer MT (2003) Contact allergy to decyl glucoside in antiseptic after body piercing. Contact Dermatitis 48:279–280

9. Allicin

CAS Registry Number [539–86–6]

Allicin is one of the major allergens in garlic (*Allium sativum* L.). It is responsible for the characteristic flavor of the bulbs, and has immunomodulating and antibacterial properties.

Suggested Reading
Bruynzeel DP (1997) Bulb dermatitis. Dermatological problems in the flower bulb industries. Contact Dermatitis 37:70–77
Lamminpää A, Estlander T, Jolanki R, Kanerva L (1996) Occupational allergic contact dermatitis caused by decorative plants. Contact Dermatitis 34:330–335
Papageorgiou C, Corbet JP, Menezes-Brandao F, Pecegueiro M, Benezra C (1983) Allergic contact dermatitis to garlic (*Allium sativum* L.). Identification of the allergens: the role of mono-, di-, and tri-sulfides present in garlic. A comparative study in man and animal (guinea pig). Arch Dermatol Res 275:229–234

10. Allyl Glycidyl Ether

CAS Registry Number [106–92–3]

Allyl glycidyl ether is a monoglycidyl derivative, used as a reactive epoxy diluent for epoxy resins. As an impurity, it was considered to be the sensitizing agent in a plastic industry worker allergic to 3-glycidyloxypropyl trimethoxysilane, an epoxy silane compound used as a fixing additive in silicone and polyurethane.

Suggested Reading

Angelini G, Rigano L, Foti C, Grandolfo M, Vena GA, Bonamonte D, Soleo L, Scorpiniti AA (1996) Occupational sensitization to epoxy resin and reactive diluents in marble workers. Contact Dermatitis 35 : 11–16

Dooms-Goossens A, Bruze M, Buysse L, Fregert S, Gruvberger B, Stals H (1995) Contact allergy to allyl glycidyl ether present as an impurity in 3-glycidyloxypropyltrimethoxysilane, a fixing additive in silicone and polyurethane. Contact Dermatitis 33 : 17–19

Jolanki R, Kanerva L, Estlander T, Tarvainen K, Keskinen H, Henriks-Eckerman ML (1990) Occupational dermatoses from epoxy resin compounds. Contact Dermatitis 23 : 172–183

11. Allyl Isothiocyanate

CAS Registry Number [57–06–7]

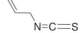

Allyl isothiocyanate is generated by enzymatic hydrolysis of the glucoside sinigrin, present in Cruciferae–Brassicaceae, mainly the oil from black mustard seed (*Brassica nigra* Koch). It may induce irritant and sometimes allergic contact dermatitis, mimicking the "tulip finger" dermatitis.

Suggested Reading

Ettlinger MG, Lundeen AJ (1956) The structures of sinigrin and sinalbin; an enzymatic rearrangement. J Ann Chem Soc 78 : 4172–4173

Lerbaek A, Chandra Rastogi S, Menné T (2004) Allergic contact dermatitis from allyl isothiocyanate in a Danish cohort of 259 selected patients. Contact Dermatitis 51 : 79–83

12. Allylpropyldisulfide

CAS Registry Number [2179–59–1]

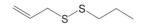

With allicin and diallyl sulfide, allylpropyldisulfide is one of the allergens in garlic (*Allium sativum* L.).

Suggested Reading
Bruynzeel DP (1997) Bulb dermatitis. Dermatological problems in the
  flower bulb industries. Contact Dermatitis 37:70–77

13. Alprenolol

CAS Registry Number
[13655–52–2]

Occupational cases of contact dermatitis were reported in the
pharmaceutical industry.

Suggested Reading
Ekenvall L, Forsbeck M (1978) Contact eczema produced by α-adrenergic
  blocking agent (Alprenolol). Contact Dermatitis 4:190–194

14. Amethocaine

Pantocaine, Tetracaine

CAS Registry Number
[136–47–0]

· HCl

Amethocaine is a local anesthetic used in dental surgery. It was
reported as an agent of contact dermatitis in dentists or dental
nurses, and in ophthalmologists.

Suggested Reading
Berova N, Stranky L, Krasteva M (1990) Studies on contact dermatitis in
  stomatological staff. Dermatol Monatschr 176:15–18
Condé-Salazar L, Llinas MG, Guimaraens D, Romero L (1988) Occupation-
  al allergic contact dermatitis from amethocaine. Contact Dermatitis
  19:69–70
Rebandel P, Rudzki E (1986) Occupational contact sensitivity in oculists.
  Contact Dermatitis 15:92

15. *p*-Amino-*N,N*-Diethylaniline Sulfate

1,4-Benzenediamine, *N,N-Diethyl-para*-Phenylenediamine Sulfate

CAS Registry Number [6065–27–6]

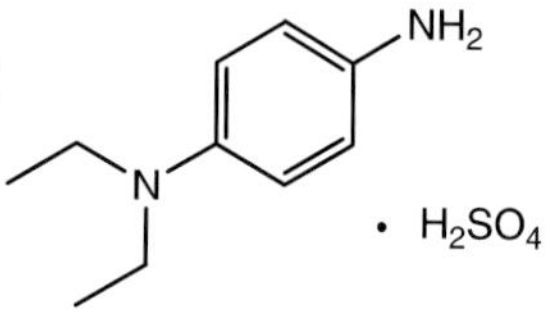

This color developer can induce sensitization in photographers.

Suggested Reading

Aguirre A, Landa N, Gonzalez M, Diaz-Perez JL (1992) Allergic contact dermatitis in a photographer. Contact Dermatitis 27:340–341

16. 4-Amino-3-Nitrophenol

3-Nitro-4-Aminophenol

CAS Registry Number [610–81–1]

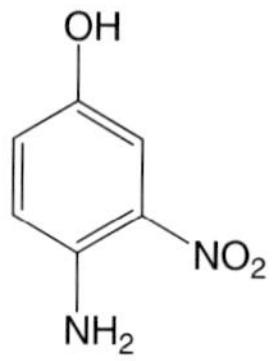

This hair dye used for semi-permanent colors seems to be a rare sensitizer.

Suggested Reading

Sánchez-Pérez J, García del Río I, Alvares Ruiz S, García Diez A (2004) Allergic contact dermatitis from direct dyes for hair coloration in hairdressers' clients. Contact Dermatitis 50:261–262

17. *p*-Aminoazobenzene

Solvent Yellow 1, C.I. 11000, Solvent Blue 7

CAS Registry Number [60–09–3]

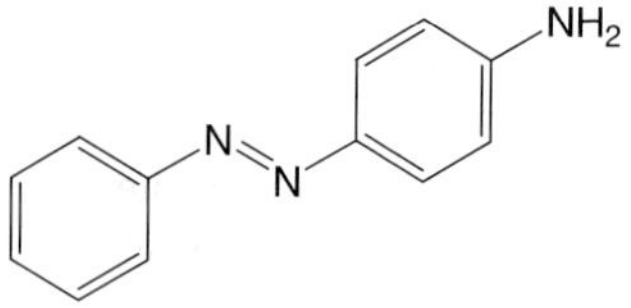

This azoic coloring can be reduced in *para*-phenylenediamine (PPD). It can be found in some semi-permanent hair dyes and patch tests are frequently positive (about 30%) in hairdressers with hand dermatitis. Because of hydrolysis of the azo bond, the detection of sensitization to *p*-aminoazobenzene may be assumed by a PPD test.

Suggested Reading

Condé-Salazar L, Baz M, Guimaraens D, Cannavo A (1995) Contact dermatitis in hairdressers: patch test results in 379 hairdressers (1980–1993). Am J Contact Dermat 6 : 19–23

18. *p*-Aminodiphenylamine (Hydrochloride)

4-Aminodiphenylamine (HCl), CI 76086 (CI 75085)

CAS Registry Number [101–54–2]
(CAS Registry Number
[2198–59–6])

(.HCl)

This substance was formerly used as a hair dye. Sensitization, when detected by patch testing, is relatively low in hairdressers.

Suggested Reading
Frosch PJ, Burrows D, Camarasa JG, Dooms-Goossens A, Ducombs G, Lahti A, Menné T, Rycroft RJG, Shaw S, White IR, Wilkinson JD (1993) Allergic reactions to a hairdresser's series: results from 9 European centres. Contact Dermatitis 28 : 180–183

19. Aminoethylethanolamine

N-(2-Hydroxyethyl)Ethylenediamine

CAS Registry Number
[111–41–1]

Aminoethylethanolamine is a component of colophony in soldering flux, which may cause contact and airborne contact dermatitis in workers in the electronic industry or in cable jointers.

Suggested Reading

Crow KD, Harman RRM, Holden H (1968) Amine-flux sensitization dermatitis in electricity cable jointers. Br J Dermatol 80:701–710

Goh CL (1985) Occupational contact dermatitis from soldering flux among workers in the electronics industry. Contact Dermatitis 13: 85–90

Goh CL, Ng SK (1987) Airborne contact dermatitis to colophony in soldering flux. Contact Dermatitis 17:89–91

20. *o*-Aminophenol

2-Aminophenol, CI 76520

CAS Registry Number [95–55–6]

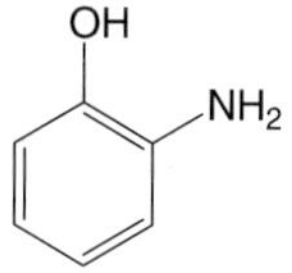

It is contained in hair dyes and can cause contact dermatitis in hairdressers and in consumers.

Suggested Reading

Matsunaga K, Hosokawa K, Suzuki M, Arima Y, Hayakawa R (1988) Occupational allergic contact dermatitis in beauticians. Contact Dermatitis 18:94–96

21. *p*-Aminophenol

4-Aminophenol, Amino-4 Hydroxybenzene, Hydroxy-4 Aniline, CI 76550

CAS Registry Number [123–30–8]

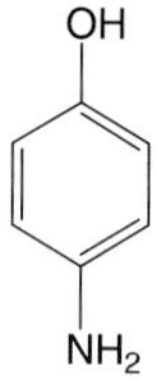

This hair dye is frequently implicated in contact dermatitis in hairdressers, in customers, or in people sensitized to *para*-phenylenediamine, by the way of "black-henna" temporary tattoos.

Suggested Reading

Guerra L, Tosti A, Bardazzi F, Pigatto P, Lisi P, Santucci B, Valsecchi R, Schena D, Angelini G, Sertoli A, Ayala F, Kokeli F (1992) Contact dermatitis in hairdressers: the Italian experience. Gruppo Italiano Ricerca Dermatiti da Contatto e Ambientali. Contact Dermatitis 26 : 101–107

Le Coz CJ, Lefebvre C, Keller F, Grosshans E (2000) Allergic contact dermatitis caused by skin painting (pseudotattooing) with black henna, a mixture of henna and p-phenylenediamine and its derivatives. Arch Dermatol 136 : 1515–1517

22. Aminophylline

Theophylline Ethylenediamine

CAS Registry Number [317–34–0]

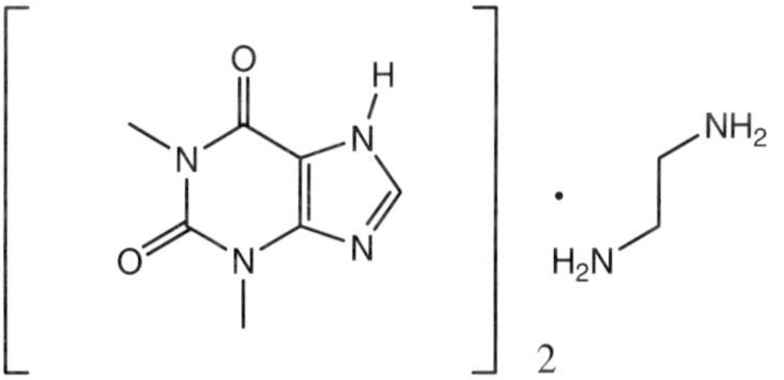

This drug is a 2 : 1 mixture of the alkaloid theophylline and ethylenediamine (see below). It caused contact dermatitis in industrial plants, in pharmacists, and in nurses. Ethylenediamine is the sensitizer and patch testing is generally positive to both ethylenediamine and aminophylline, and negative to theophylline.

Suggested Reading

Corazza M, Mantovani L, Trimurti L, Virgili A (1994) Occupational contact sensitization to ethylenediamine in a nurse. Contact Dermatitis 31 : 328–329

Dias M, Fernandes C, Pereira F, Pacheco A (1995) Occupational dermatitis from ethylenediamine. Contact Dermatitis 33 : 129–130

23. N,N-bis-(3-Aminopropyl) Dodecylamine

N-(3-Aminopropyl)-N-Dodecyl-1,3-Propanediamine

CAS Registry Number [2372–82–9]

This alkylamine is contained in detergent-disinfectants solutions for medical instruments. It is also contained in association with 3-aminopropyl dodecylamine in liquid laundry disinfectants such as Aset® aqua (Johnson Wax SpA, Rydelle).

Suggested Reading

Dibo M, Brasch J (2001) Occupational allergic contact dermatitis from N,N-bis(3-aminopropyl)dodecylamine and dimethyldid-ecylammonium chloride in two hospital staff. Contact Dermatitis 45 : 40

24. Ammonium Persulfate

Ammonium Peroxydisulfate

CAS Registry Number [317–34–0]

Persulfates are strong oxidizing agents widely used in the production of metals, textiles, photographs, cellophane, rubber, adhesive papers, foods, soaps, detergents, and hair bleaches. Ammonium persulfate is used as a hair bleaching agent. It may induce irritant dermatitis, (mainly) nonimmunologic contact urticaria, and allergic contact dermatitis and represents a major allergen in hairdressers. People reacting to ammonium persulfate also react to other persulfates such as potassium persulfate.

Suggested Reading

Frosch PJ, Burrows D, Camarasa JG, Dooms-Goossens A, Ducombs G, Lahti A, Menné T, Rycroft RJG, Shaw S, White IR, Wilkinson JD (1993)

Allergic reactions to a hairdresser's series: results from 9 European centres. Contact Dermatitis 28:180–183

Le Coz CJ, Bezard M (1999) Allergic contact cheilitis due to effervescent dental cleanser: combined responsibilities of the allergen persulfate and prosthesis porosity. Contact Dermatitis 41:268–271

Van Joost T, Roesyanto ID (1991) Sensitization to persulphates in occupational and non-occupational hand dermatitis. Contact Dermatitis 24: 376–377

25. Ammonium Thioglycolate

Ammonium Mercaptoacetate

CAS Registry Number [5421–46–5]

$$HS\frown CO_2^{\ominus} \cdot NH_4^{\oplus}$$

This substance is contained in "basic" permanent waves solutions and causes contact dermatitis in hairdressers.

Suggested Reading

Frosch PJ, Burrows D, Camarasa JG, Dooms-Goossens A, Ducombs G, Lahti A, Menné T, Rycroft RJG, Shaw S, White IR, Wilkinson JD (19939 Allergic reactions to a hairdresser's series: results from 9 European centres. Contact Dermatitis 28:180–183

Guerra L, Tosti A, Bardazzi F, Pigatto P, Lisi P, Santucci B, Valsecchi R, Schena D, Angelini G, Sertoli A, Ayala F, Kokeli F (1992) Contact dermatitis in hairdressers: the Italian experience. Gruppo Italiano Ricerca Dermatiti da Contatto e Ambientali. Contact Dermatitis 26:101–107

26. Amoxicillin

CAS Registry Number
[26787–78–0]

Amoxicillin Trihydrate

CAS Registry Number
[61336–70–7]

Amoxicillin Sodium Salt

CAS Registry Number [34642–77–8]

Amoxicillin is both a topical and a systemic sensitizer. Topical sensitization occurs in healthcare workers. Systemic drug reactions are frequent, such as urticaria, maculo-papular rashes, baboon syndrome, acute generalized exanthematous pustulosis, or even toxic epidermal necrosis. Cross-reactivity is common with ampicillin, and can occur with other penicillins.

Suggested Reading
Gamboa P, Jauregui I, Urrutia I (1995) Occupational sensitization to amino-penicillins with oral tolerance to penicillin V. Contact Dermatitis 32 : 48–49
Rudzki E, Rebandel P (1991) Hypersensitivity to semisynthetic penicillins but not to natural penicillin. Contact Dermatitis 25 : 192

27. Ampicillin

CAS Registry Number [69–53–4]

Ampicillin Trihydrate

CAS Registry Number [7177–48–2]

Ampicillin Sodium Salt

CAS Registry Number [69–52–3]

Ampicillin caused contact dermatitis in a nurse also sensitized to amoxicillin (with tolerance to oral phenoxymethylpenicillin), and in a pharmaceutical factory worker. Systemic drug reactions are common. Cross-reactivity is regular with ampicillin, and can occur with other penicillins.

Suggested Reading
Gamboa P, Jauregui I, Urrutia I (1995) Occupational sensitization to amino-penicillins with oral tolerance to penicillin V. Contact Dermatitis 32 : 48–49
Rudzki E, Rebandel P (1991) Hypersensitivity to semisynthetic penicillins but not to natural penicillin. Contact Dermatitis 25 : 192

28. Amprolium (Hydrochloride)

CAS Registry Number [121–25–5]
(CAS Registry Number [137–88–2])

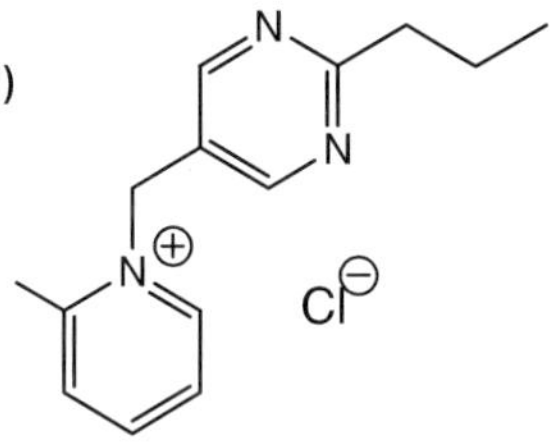

Amprolium is an antiprotozoal agent used for the prevention of coccidiosis in poultry.

Suggested Reading

Mancuso G, Staffa M, Errani A, Berdondini RM, Fabbri P (1990) Occupational dermatitis in animal feed mill workers. Contact Dermatitis 22: 37–41

29. Amyl Cinnamyl Alcohol

2-Pentyl-3-Phenylprop-2-en-1-ol, Pentyl-Cinnamic Alcohol, α-Amyl-Cinnamic Alcohol, Buxinol

CAS Registry number [101–85–9]

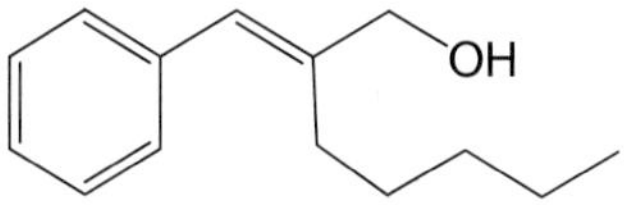

This scented molecule is very close to α-amyl-cinnamic aldehyde. Its presence is indicated by name in cosmetics within the EU.

Suggested Reading

Rastogi SC, Johansen JD, Menné T (1996) Natural ingredients based cosmetics. Content of selected fragrance sensitizers. Contact Dermatitis 34: 423–426

30. Amylcinnamaldehyde

α-Amyl Cinnamic Aldehyde, Ammylcinnamal,
2-Benzylideneheptanal,
2-Pentylcinnamaldehyde, Jasminal

CAS Registry Number [122–40–7]

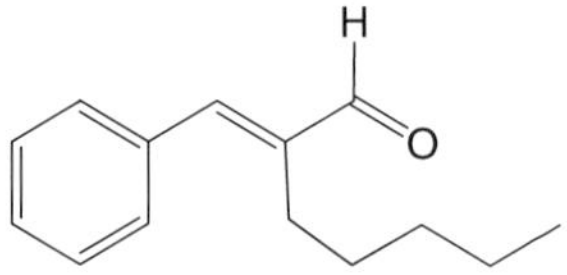

α-Amyl cinnamic aldehyde is an oxidation product of amylcinnamic alcohol, a sensitizing fragrance and one component of the "fragrance mix". It can also be a sensitizer in bakers. It has to be mentioned by name in cosmetics within the EU.

Suggested Reading
Nethercott JR, Holness DL (1989) Occupational dermatitis in food handlers and bakers. J Am Acad Dermatol 21:485–490

31. Anacardic Acids

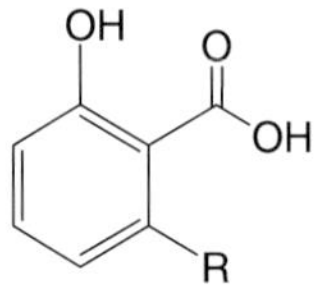

Anacardic acids are mixture of several analog molecules with alkyl chain (-R) of 13, 15, 17, or 19 carbons, and 0 to 3 unsaturations. They are the main cashew nut shell liquid component with cardol and can cause contact dermatitis in cashew nut workers.

Suggested Reading
Diogenes MJN, de Morais SM, Carvalho FF (1996) Contact dermatitis among cashew nut workers. Contact Dermatitis 35:114–115

32. Anethole

1-Methoxy-4-(1-Propenyl)-Benzene

CAS Registry Number [104–46–1]

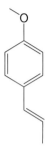

Anethole is the main component of anise, star anise, and fennel oils. It is used in perfumes, in the food and cosmetic industries (toothpastes), in bleaching colors, photography, and as an embedding material.

Suggested Reading

Garcia-Bravo B, Pérez Bernal A, Garcia-Hernandez MJ, Camacho F (1997) Occupational contact dermatitis from anethole in food handlers. Contact Dermatitis 37:38

33. Anisyl Alcohol

4-Methoxybenzyl Alcohol, Methoxybenzenemethanol, Anise Alcohol

CAS Registry Number [105–13–5]

Blend of *o*-, *m*-, and *p*-Methoxybenzyl Alcohol

CAS Registry number [1331–81–3]

As a fragrance allergen, anisyl alcohol has to be mentioned by name in cosmetics within the EU.

Suggested Reading
Budavari S, O'Neil MJ, Smith A, Heckelman PE, Kinneary JF (eds) (1996) The Merck Index, 12th edn. Merck, Whitehouse Station, N.J., USA

34. Antimony Trioxide

CAS Registry Number [1309–64–4] Sb_2O_3

This hard shiny metal is often alloyed to other elements. It is used in various industrial fields such as batteries, printing machines, bearing, textile, and ceramics. It caused positive patch test reactions in two workers in the ceramics industry.

Suggested Reading
Motolese A, Truzzi M, Giannini A, Seidenari S (1995) Contact dermatitis and contact sensitization among enamellers and decorators in the ceramics industry. Contact Dermatitis 28 : 59–62

35. Arsenic and Arsenic Salts (Sodium Arsenate)

**CAS Registry Number [7440–38–2]
and CAS Registry Number [7778–43–0]**

As AsO_4H_2Na

Arsenic salts are sensitizers, but most often irritants. They are used in copper or gold extraction, glass, feeds, weedkillers, insecticides, and ceramics. A recent case was reported in a crystal factory worker with positive patch tests to sodium arsenate.

Suggested Reading
Barbaud A, Mougeolle JM, Schmutz JL (1995) Contact hypersensitivity to arsenic in a crystal factory worker. Contact Dermatitis 33 : 272–273

36. Articaine (Hydrochloride)

Carticaine (Hydrochloride)

CAS Registry Number [23964–58–1]
(CAS Registry Number [23964–57–0])

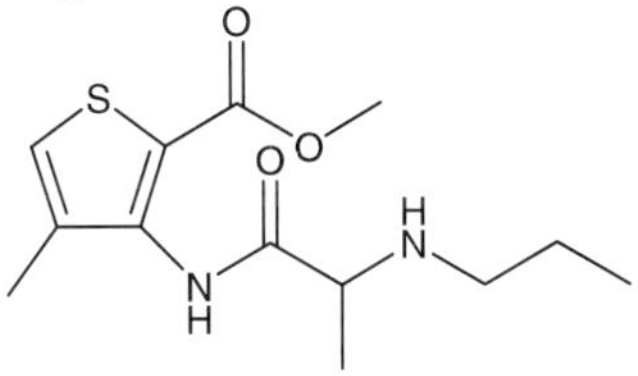

This local amide-type anesthetic is seldom reported as allergenic even in patients sensitized to other amide-type molecules like lidocaine, prilocaine, mepivacaine or bupivacaine.

Suggested Reading

Duque S, Fernandez L (2004) Delayed-type hypersensitivity to amide local anaesthetics. Allergol Immunopathol (Madr) 32:233–234

37. Atranol

2,6-Dihydroxy-4-Methyl-Benzaldehyde

CAS Registry number [526–37–4]

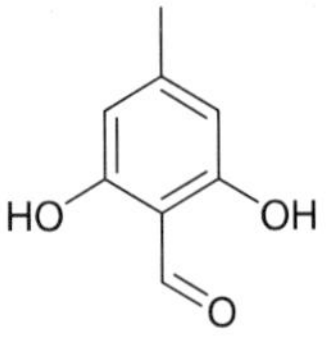

Atranol has been identified as a potent and frequent allergen, occurring from the fragrance material oak-moss absolute, which is of botanical origin.

Suggested Reading

Johansen JD, Andersen KE, Svedman C, Bruze M, Bernard G, Giménez-Arnau E, Rastogi SC, Lepoittevin JP, Menné T (2003) Chloroatranol, an extremely potent allergen hidden in perfumes: a dose response elicitation study. Contact Dermatitis 49:180–184

Rastogi SC, Bossi R, Johansen JD, Menné T, Bernard G, Giménez-Arnau E, Lepoittevin P (2004) Content of oak moss allergens atranol and chloroatranol in perfumes and similar products. Contact Dermatitis 50:367–370

38. Azaperone

4′-Fluoro-4-[4-(2-Pyridyl)-1-Piperazininyl]Butyrophenone

CAS Registry Number [1649–18–9]

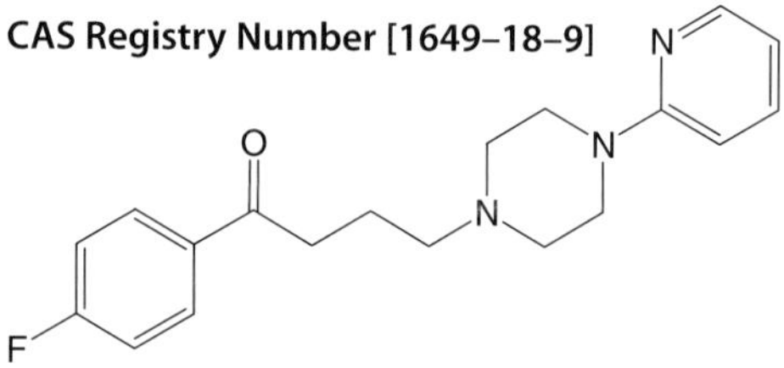

Azaperone is a sedative used in veterinary medicine, to avoid mortality of pigs during transportation. This alternative substance to chlorpromazine is a sensitizer and a photosensitizer.

Suggested Reading

Brasch J, Hessler HJ, Christophers E (1991) Occupational (photo)allergic contact dermatitis from azaperone in a piglet dealer. Contact Dermatitis 25:258–259

39. Azathioprine

6-(1-Methyl-4-Nitroimidazol-5-ylthio)Purine

CAS Registry Number [446–86–6]

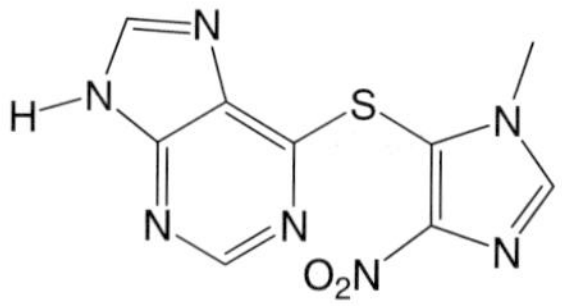

This immunosuppressive and antineoplastic drug is derived from 6-mercaptopurine. It caused allergic contact dermatitis in a mother crushing tablets for her leukemic son, and occupational dermatitis in a pharmaceutical reconditioner of old tablet packaging machines, and in a production mechanic working in packaging for a pharmaceutical company.

Suggested Reading

Burden AD, Beck MH (1992) Contact hypersensitivity to azathioprine. Contact Dermatitis 27:329–330

Lauerma A, Koivuluhta M, Alenius H (2001) Recalcitrant allergic contact dermatitis from azathioprine tablets. Contact Dermatitis 44:129

Soni BP, Sherertz EF (1996) Allergic contact dermatitis from azathioprine. Am J Contact Dermat 7:116–117

40. Basic Red 22

Synacril Red 3B

CAS Registry Number
[12221–52–2]

This monoazoic dye was reported as allergenic in a PPD-free hair coloring mousse.

Suggested Reading

Salim A, Orton D, Shaw S (2001) Allergic contact dermatitis from Basic Red 22 in a hair-colouring mousse. Contact Dermatitis 45:123

41. Basic Red 46

CAS Registry Number
[12221–69–1]

This monoazoic textile dye seems to be an important cause of foot dermatitis, being a frequent allergen in acrylic socks. It caused contact dermatitis in two workers in the textile industry.

Suggested Reading

Opie J, Lee A, Frowen K, Fewings J, Nixon R (2003) Foot dermatitis caused by the textile dye Basic Red 46 in acrylic blend socks. Contact Dermatitis 49:297–303

Soni BP, Sherertz EF (1996) Contact dermatitis in the textile industry: a review of 72 patients. Am J Contact Dermat 7:226–230

42. Befunolol

CAS Registry Number [39552-01-7]

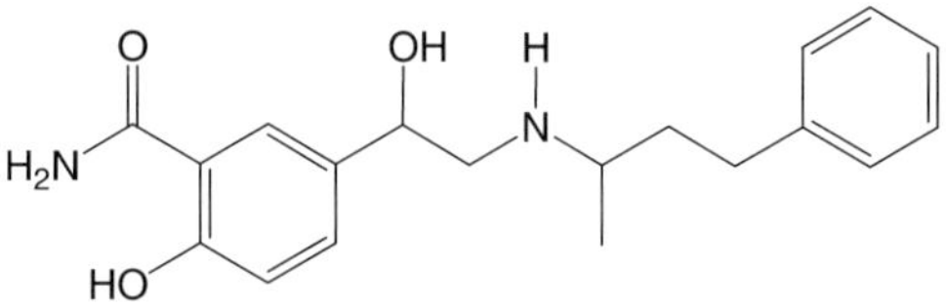

Befunolol was implicated in allergic contact dermatitis due to beta-blocker agents in eye-drops.

Suggested Reading

Giordano-Labadie F, Lepoittevin JP, Calix I, Bazex J (1997) Allergie de contact aux β-bloqueurs des collyres: allergie croisée? Ann Dermatol Venereol 124:322–324

43. Benomyl

CAS Registry Number [17804-35-2]

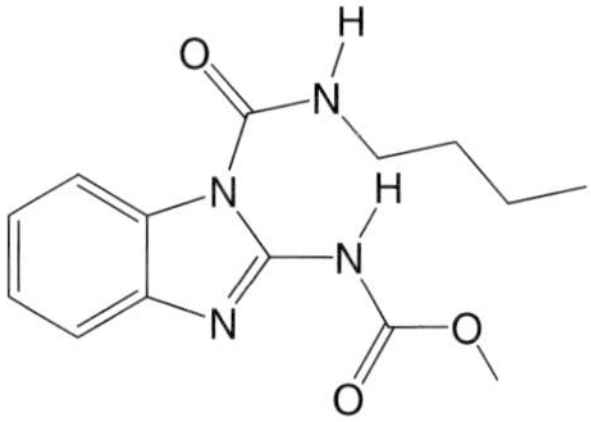

Benomyl is a fungicide, derived from benzimidazole. Cases of sensitization were reported in horticulturists and florists. It is however, at most, a weak sensitizer, with possible false-positive patch reactions, or with cross-reactions after previous exposure to other fungicides.

Suggested Reading

Jung HD, Honemann W, Kloth C, Lubbe D, Pambor M, Quednow C, Ratz KH, Rothe A, Tarnick M (1989) Kontaktekzem durch Pestizide in der Deutschen Demokratischen Republik. Dermatol Monats 175:203–214

Larsen AI, Larsen A, Jepsen JR, Jorgensen R (1990) Contact allergy to the fungicide benomyl? Contact Dermatitis 22:278–281

O'Malley M, Rodriguez P, Maibach HI (1995) Pesticide patch testing: California nursery workers and controls. Contact Dermatitis 32:61–62

44. Benzalkonium Chloride

CAS Registry Number [8001–54–5]

This quaternary ammonium cationic surfactant is a mixture of alkyl, dimethyl, and benzyl ammonium chlorides (-R). It is an irritant rather than a sensitizer, but may cause allergic contact dermatitis from creams, detergents/antiseptics, ophthalmic preparations, and in nursing, veterinary, dental, and medical personnel. Its presence was observed in plaster of Paris.

Suggested Reading

Basketter DA, Marriott M, Gilmour NJ, White IR (2004) Strong irritants masquerading as skin allergens: the case of benzalkonium chloride. Contact Dermatitis 50 : 213–217

Corazza M, Virgili A (1993) Airborne allergic contact dermatitis from benzalkonium chloride. Contact Dermatitis 28 : 195–196

Klein GF, Sepp N, Fritsch P (1991) Allergic reactions to benzalkonium chloride? Do the use test! Contact Dermatitis 25 : 269–270

Stanford D, Georgouras K (1996) Allergic contact dermatitis from benzalkonium chloride in plaster of Paris. Contact Dermatitis 35 : 371–372

45. Benzisothiazolone

1,2-Benzisothiazolin-3-one, BIT, Proxan, Proxel PL

CAS Registry Number [2634–33–5]

BIT, both an irritant and a skin sensitizer, is widely used in industry as a preservative in water-based solutions such as pastes, paints, and cutting oils. Occupational dermatitis has been reported mainly due to cutting fluids and greases, in paint manufacturers, pottery mold-makers, in acrylic emulsions manufacturers, in plumber, printers and lithoprinters, paper makers, analytical laboratory, rubber factory, and in employees manufacturing air fresheners.

Suggested Reading

Burden AD, O'Driscoll JB, Page FC, Beck MH (1994) Contact hypersensitivity to a new isothiazolinone. Contact Dermatitis 30:179–180

Chew AL, Maibach H (1997) 1,2-Benzisothiazolin-3-one (Proxel®): irritant or allergen? A clinical study and literature review. Contact Dermatitis 36:131–136

Dias M, Lamarao P, Vale T (1992) Occupational contact allergy to 1,2-benzisothiazolin-3-one in the manufacture of air fresheners. Contact Dermatitis 27:205–206

Greig DE (1991) Another isothiazolinone source. Contact Dermatitis 25:201–202

Sanz-Gallén P, Planas J, Martinez P, Giménez-Arnau JM (1992) Allergic contact dermatitis due to 1,2-benzisothiazolin-3-one in paint manufacture. Contact Dermatitis 27:271–272

46. Benzophenones

Benzophenone (BZP), and substituted BZP numbered 1–12, trade mark Uvinul®, are photo-screen agents widely used in sunscreens and in cosmetics, such as "anti-aging" creams and hair sprays and shampoos, paints and plastics. The hypolipemiant drug fenofibrate is also a substituted benzophenone.

Benzophenone, Unsubstituted
CAS Registry Number [119–61–9]

Unsubstituted benzophenone is largely used in chemical applications. It acts as a marker for photoallergy to ketoprofen.

Benzophenone 1
Benzoresorcinol, Uvinul 400
CAS Registry Number [131–56–6]

BZP-1 is used in paints, plastics and nail varnishes, for example.

Benzophenone-2
2,2′,4,4′-Tetrahydroxybenzophenone
CAS Registry Number [131–55–5]

BZP-2 is widely used in perfumes to prevent their degradation due to light. It can cause allergic contact dermatitis.

Benzophenone-3

Oxybenzone

CAS Registry Number [131–57–7]

BZP-3 is used as a direct sunscreen agent, and in anti-aging creams. Allergic reactions have been reported. Cross reactivity is expected in an average of one in four patients photoallergic to ketoprofen.

Benzophenone-4

Sulisobenzone

CAS Registry Number [4065–45–6]

BZP-4 is widely used in cosmetics, particularly shampoos and hair products. Cross reactivity is rarely expected in patients photoallergic to ketoprofen.

Benzophenone-10

Mexenone

CAS Registry Number [1641–17–4]

BZP-10 is exceptionally positive in ketoprofen-photosensitive patients.

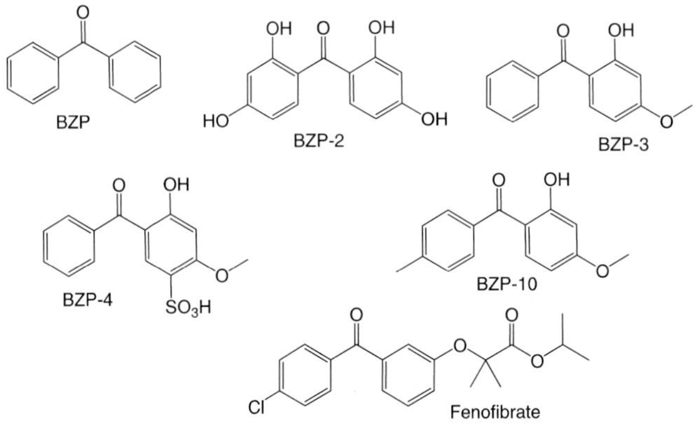

Suggested Reading

Alanko K, Jolanki R, Estlander T, Kanerva L (2001) Occupational allergic contact dermatitis from benzophenone-4 in hair-care products. Contact Dermatitis 44:188

Collins P, Ferguson J (1994) Photoallergic contact dermatitis to oxybenzone. Br J Dermatol 131:124–129

Guin JD (2000) Eyelid dermatitis from benzophenone used in nail enhancement. Contact Dermatitis 43:308–309

Jacobs MC (1998) Contact allergy to benzophenone-2 in toilet water. Contact Dermatitis 39:42

Knobler E, Almeida L, Ruzkowski AM, Held J, Harber L, DeLeo V (1989) Photoallergy to benzophenone. Arch Dermatol 125:801–804

Le Coz CJ, Bottlaender A, Scrivener JN, Santinelli F, Cribier BJ, Heid E, Grosshans EM (1998) Photocontact dermatitis from ketoprofen and tiaprofenic acid: cross-reactivity study in 12 consecutive patients. Contact Dermatitis 38:245–252

Matthieu L, Meuleman L, van Hecke E, Blondeel A, Dezfoulian B, Constandt L, Goossens A (2004) Contact and photocontact allergy to ketoprofen. The Belgian experience. Contact Dermatitis 50:238–241

Ramsay DL, Cohen HJ, Baer RL (1972) Allergic reaction to benzophenone. Simultaneous occurrence of urticarial and contact sensitivities. Arch Dermatol 105:906–908

47. Benzoyl Peroxide

CAS Registry Number [94–36–0]

Benzoyl peroxide is an oxidizing agent widely employed in acne topical therapy. It is also used as a polymerization catalyst of dental or industrial plastics, as a decolorizing agent of flours, oils, fats, and waxes. Irritant or allergic dermatitis may affect workers in the electronics and plastics (epoxy resins and catalysts) industries, electricians, ceramic workers, dentists and dental technicians, laboratory technicians, bakers, and acne patients. As it was contained in candles, it also induced contact dermatitis in a sacristan. Patch tests may be irritant.

Suggested Reading

Balato N, Lembo G, Cuccurullo FM, Patruno C, Nappa P, Ayala F (1996) Acne and allergic contact dermatitis. Contact Dermatitis 34: 68–69

Bonnekoh B, Merk H (1991) Airborne allergic contact dermatitis from benzoyl peroxyde as a bleaching agent of candle wax. Contact Dermatitis 24:367–368

Quirce S, Olaguibel JM, Garcia BE, Tabar AI (1993) Occupational airborne contact dermatitis due to benzoyl peroxide. Contact Dermatitis 29: 165–166

Rustemeyer T, Frosch PJ (1996) Occupational skin diseases in dental laboratory technicians. (I). Clinical picture and causative factors. Contact Dermatitis 34:125–133

48. Benzydamine Hydrochloride

CAS Registry Number [132-69-4]

· HCl

It is a nonsteroidal anti-inflammatory drug used both topically and systemically. It has been reported as a sensitizer and a photosensitizer.

Suggested Reading

Foti C, Vena GA, Angelini G (1992) Occupational contact allergy to benzydamine hydrochloride. Contact Dermatitis 27:328–329

Lasa Elgezua O, Egino Gorrotxategi P, Gardeazabal García J, Ratón Nieto JA, Díaz Pérez JL (2004) Photoallergic hand eczema due to benzydamine. Eur J Dermatol 14:69–70

49. Benzyl Alcohol

CAS Registry Number [100-51-6]

Benzyl alcohol is mainly a preservative, mostly used in topical antimycotic or corticosteroid ointments. It is also a component catalyst for epoxy resins, and is contained in the color developer C-22. As a fragrance allergen, it has to be mentioned by name in cosmetics within the EU.

Suggested Reading

Lodi A, Mancini LL, Pozzi M, Chiarelli G, Crosti C (1993) Occupational airborne allergic contact dermatitis in parquet layers. Contact Dermatitis 29 : 281–282

Scheman AJ, Katta R (1997) Photographic allergens: an update. Contact Dermatitis 37 : 130

Sestini S, Mori M, Francalanci S (2004) Allergic contact dermatitis from benzyl alcohol in multiple medicaments. Contact Dermatitis 50 : 316–317

50. Benzyl Benzoate

Benzoic Acid Phenylmethyl Ester

CAS Registry Number [120–51–4]

Benzyl benzoate is the ester of benzyl alcohol and benzoic acid. It is contained in *Myroxylon pereirae* and Tolu balsam. It is used in acaricide preparations against *Sarcoptes scabiei* or as a pediculicide. Direct contact may cause skin irritation but rarely allergic contact dermatitis. As a fragrance allergen, benzyl benzoate has to be mentioned by name in EU cosmetics.

Suggested Reading

Meneghini CL, Vena GA, Angelini G (1982) Contact dermatitis to scabicides. Contact Dermatitis 8 : 285–286

51. Benzyl Salicylate

Benzyl-o-Hydroxybenzoate, 2-Hydroxybenzoic Acid Phenylmethyl Ester

CAS Registry Number [118–58–1]

Benzyl salicylate is used as fixer in perfumery and in sunscreen preparations. As a (weak) perfume sensitizer, it has to be listed by name in cosmetic preparations in the EU.

Suggested Reading
Larsen W, Nakayama H, Lindberg M, Fischer T, Elsner P, Burrows D, Jordan W, Shaw S, Wilkinson J, Marks J Jr, Sugawara M, Nethercott J (1996) Fragrance contact dermatitis: a worldwide multicenter investigation (Part I). Am J Contact Dermat 7:77–83

52. Benzylpenicillin

Penicillin G

CAS Registry Number
[61–33–6]

Benzyl penicillin is actually used only intravenously. It was formerly a frequent cause of contact allergy in healthcare workers. Facial contact dermatitis was recently reported in a nurse.

Suggested Reading
Pecegueiro M (1990) Occupational contact dermatitis from penicillin. Contact Dermatitis 23:190–191

53. BHA

Butylated Hydroxyanisole

CAS Registry Number
[25013–16–5]

BHA is an antioxidant widely used in cosmetics and food. Contained in pastry, it can induce sensitization in caterers.

Suggested Reading

Acciai MC, Brusi C, Francalanci Giorgini S, Sertoli A (1993) Allergic contact dermatitis in caterers. Contact Dermatitis 28:48

54. BHT

Butylated Hydroxytoluene, 2,6-di-(tert-Butyl)-p-Cresol

CAS Registry Number [128–37–0]

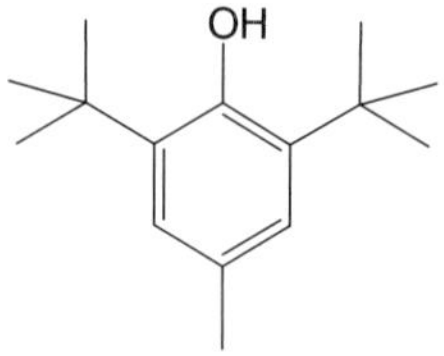

This antioxidant is contained in food, adhesive glues, industrial oils and greases, including cutting fluids. Sensitization seems very rare.

Suggested Reading

Flyvholm MA, Menné T (1990) Sensitizing risk of butylated hydroxytoluene based on exposure and effect data. Contact Dermatitis 23:341–345

55. Bioban CS-1135

3,4-Dimethyloxazolidine + 3,4,4-Trimethyloxazolidine

CAS Registry Number [81099–36–7]
(CAS Registry Number [51200–87–4] +
CAS Registry Number [75673–43–7])

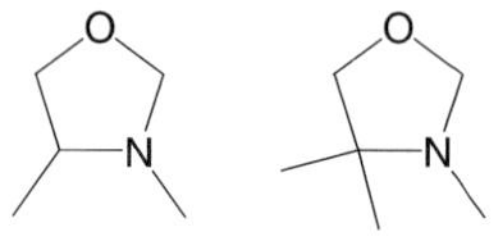

Bioban® CS-1135 is the trade name for the two compounds 3,4-dimethyloxazolidine (74.8%) and 3,4,4-trimethyloxazolidine (2.5%). It is a formaldehyde releaser used as a preservative in latex paints and emulsions, and in cooling fluids. Dimethyl oxazolidine is found in some cosmetics. Bioban® CS-1135 can be a sensitizer per se, in patients without formaldehyde allergy.

Suggested Reading

Brinkmeier T, Geier J, Lepoittevin JP, Frosch PJ (2002) Patch test reactions to Biobans in metalworkers are often weak and not reproducible. Contact Dermatitis 47:27–31

Kanerva L, Estlander T, Jolanki R (1994) Occupational allergic contact dermatitis caused by thiourea compounds. Contact Dermatitis 31: 242–248

56. Bioban® CS-1246

Oxazolidine, 5-Ethyl-1-aza-3,7-Dioxa-Bicyclo-3,3,0 Octane

CAS Registry Number [7747–35–5], [504–76–7]

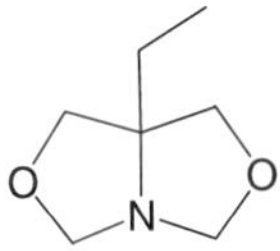

Bioban® CS-1246 is a relatively old formaldehyde releaser, used in cutting oils. Bioban® CS-1248 is a mixture of Bioban® CS-1246 and Bioban® P-1487.

Suggested Reading

Brinkmeier T, Geier J, Lepoittevin JP, Frosch PJ (2002) Patch test reactions to Biobans in metalworkers are often weak and not reproducible. Contact Dermatitis 47:27–31

57. Bioban® P-1487

4-(2-Nitrobutyl)Morpholine + 4,4′-(2-Ethyl-2-Nitrodimethylene)Dimorpholine

CAS Registry Number [37304–88–4]
(CAS Registry Number [2224–44–4] +
CAS Registry Number [1854–23–5]

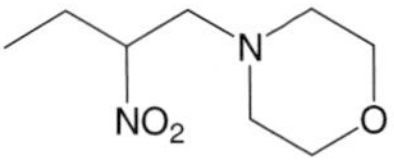

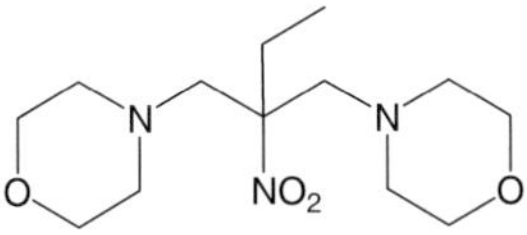

Bioban® P-1487 is a mixture of 4-(2-nitrobutyl)morpholine CAS Registry Number [2224–44–4] 70%, and 4,4′-(2-ethyl-2-nitrodimethylene)dimorpholine or 4,4'-(2-ethyl-2-nitro-1,3-propane-diyl)-bis-morpholine CAS Registry Number [1854–23–5] 20%. Both ingredients can be the sensitizers. It is used as a preservative in metalworking cutting fluids. Bioban® CS-1248 is a mixture of Bioban® CS-1246 and Bioban® P-1487.

Suggested Reading

Brinkmeier T, Geier J, Lepoittevin JP, Frosch PJ (2002) Patch test reactions to Biobans in metalworkers are often weak and not reproducible. Contact Dermatitis 47:27–31

Gruvberger B, Bruze M, Zimerson E (1996) Contact allergy to the active ingredients of Bioban P 1487. Contact Dermatitis 35:141–145

Niklasson B, Björkner B, Sundberg K (1993) Contact allergy to a fatty acid ester component of cutting fluids. Contact Dermatitis 28:265–267

58. Bisphenol A

Diphenylolpropane, Isopropylidene Diphenol

CAS Registry Number
[80–05–7]

Bisphenol A is used with epichlorhydrin for the synthesis of epoxy resins bisphenol-A type, for unsaturated polyester and polycarbonate resins, and epoxy di(meth)acrylates. In epoxy resins, it leads to bisphenol-A diglycidyl ether, which is the monomer of bisphenol-A-based epoxy resins. Reports of bisphenol-A sensitization are rare and concern workers at epoxy resin plants, after contact with fiber glass, semi-synthetic waxes, footwear, and dental materials. It is also a possible sensitizer in vinyl gloves.

Suggested Reading

Jolanki R, Kanerva L, Estlander T (1995) Occupational allergic contact dermatitis caused by epoxy diacrylate in ultraviolet-light-cured paint, and bisphenol A in dental composite resin. Contact Dermatitis 33:94–99

Matthieu L, Godoi AFL, Lambert J, van Grieken R (2004) Occupational allergic contact dermatitis from bisphenol A in vinyl gloves. Contact Dermatitis 49:281–283

Van Jost T, Roesyanto ID, Satyawan I (1990) Occupational sensitization to epichlorhydrin (ECH) and bisphenol-A during the manufacture of epoxy resin. Contact Dermatitis 22:125–126

59. Bisphenol A Diglycidyl Ether (DGEBA)

BADGE

CAS Registry Number [1675–54–3]

Most epoxy resins result from polymerization of bisphenol A diglycidyl ether (BADGE). Delayed hypersensitivity is caused by the low-molecular-weight monomer BADGE (Mol. Wt. 340 g/mol), the dimer having much a lower sensitization power. This allergen caused contact dermatitis in six workers in a plant producing printed circuits boards made of copper sheets and fiber glass fabric impregnated with a brominated epoxy resin. It can be contained in adhesives.

Suggested Reading

Bruze M, Almgren G (1989) Occupational dermatoses in workers exposed to epoxy-impregnated fiberglass fabric. Dermatosen 37:171–176

Bruze M, Edenholm M, Engenström K, Svensson G (1996) Occupational dermatoses in a Swedish aircraft plant. Contact Dermatitis 34:336–340

Hansson C (1994) Determination of monomers in epoxy resin hardened at elevated temperatures. Contact Dermatitis 31:333–334

60. *o-p′*-Bisphenol F and *p-p′*-Bisphenol F

2,4′-Dihydroxy-Diphenylmethane and 4-4′-Dihydroxy-Diphenylmethane

CAS Registry Number [2467–03–0] and CAS Registry Number [620–92–8]

o-p′-Bisphenol F and *p-p′*-bisphenol F are allergenic components of phenol-formaldehyde resins resol-type.

Suggested Reading
Bruze M, Fregert S, Zimerson E (1985) Contact allergy to phenol-formal-
    dehyde resins. Contact Dermatitis 12:81–86

61. Bisphenol F Diglycidyl Ether (DGEBF)

1. *p, p'*-Diglycidyl Ether of Bisphenol F

CAS Registry Number [2095–03–6]

2. *o,p'*-Diglycidyl Ether of Bisphenol F

CAS Registry Number [57469–08–5]

3. *o,o'*-Diglycidyl Ether of Bisphenol F

CAS Registry Number [39817–09–9], [54208–63–8]

Epoxy resins based on Bisphenol F, also called phenolic Novolac,
contain bisphenol F diglycidyl ether, which has three sensitizing
isomers. DGEBF has a greater resistance than DGEBA. Contact
allergy to bisphenol-F-based epoxy resins is rarer than that due to
bisphenol-A-based resins, and is frequently acquired with flooring
materials and putty.

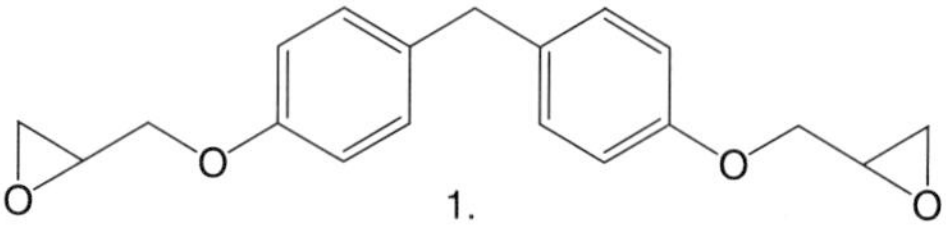

1.

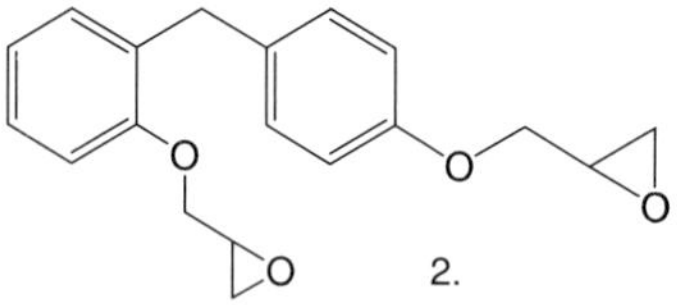

2.

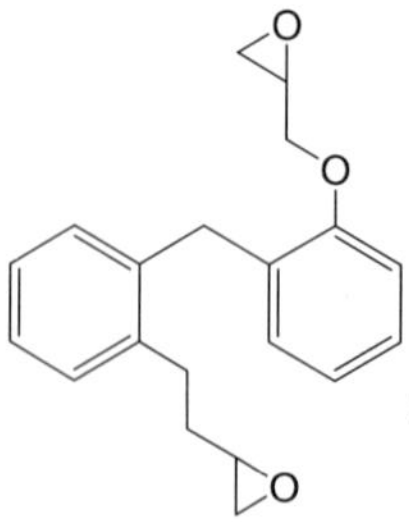

3.

Suggested Reading

Bruze M, Edenholm M, Engenström K, Svensson G (1996) Occupational dermatoses in a Swedish aircraft plant. Contact Dermatitis 34:336–340

Pontén A, Bruze M (2001) Contact allergy to epoxy resin based on diglycidyl ether of Bisphenol F. Contact Dermatitis 44:98–99

Pontén A, Zimerson E, Bruze M (2004) Contact allergy to the isomers of diglycidyl ether of bisphenol F. Acta Derm Venereol (Stockh) 84:12–17

62. Brominated Epoxy Resin

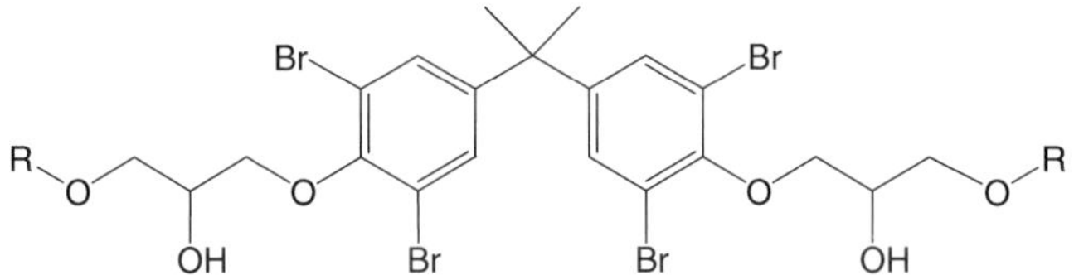

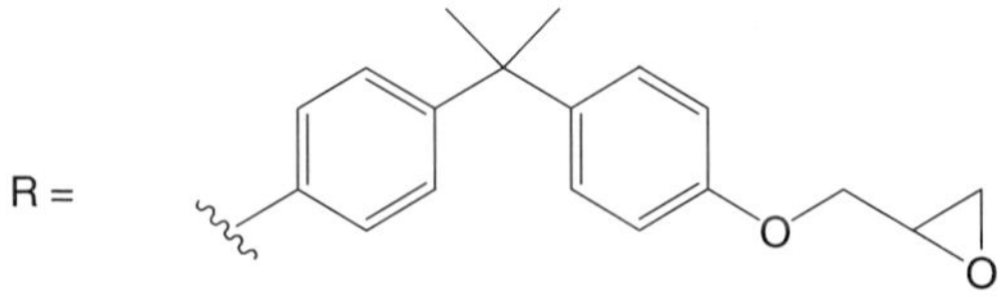

As a component of nondiglycidyl ether of bisphenol A epoxy resins, brominated epoxy resin caused contact dermatitis in a cleaner of worksites in a condenser factory, where condensers were filled with a mixture made of an epoxy resin.

Suggested Reading

Kanerva L, Jolanki R, Estlander T (1991) Allergic contact dermatitis from non-diglycidyl-ether-of-bisphenol-A epoxy resins. Contact Dermatitis 24:293–300

63. 1-Bromo-3-Chloro-5,5-Dimethylhydantoin

Di-Halo, 1-Bromo-3-Chloro-5,5-Dimethyl-2,4-Imidazolidinedione, Agribrom, Slimicide C 77P

CAS Registry Number [16079–88–2]

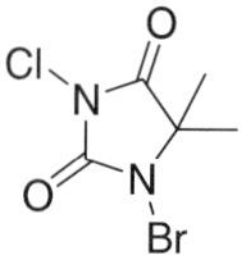

This chlorinated and brominated product is employed in agriculture as a fungicide, for wood preservation. When used to sanitize pools and spas, releasing both chlorine and bromine derivatives, it can induce irritant or allergic contact dermatitis.

Suggested Reading

Rycroft RJG, Penny PT (1983) Dermatoses associated with brominated swimming pools. Br Med J (Clin Res Ed) 287 : 462

Sasseville D, Moreau L (2004) Contact allergy to 1-bromo-3chloro-5, 5-dimethylhydantoin in spa water. Contact Dermatitis 50 : 323–324

64. Bromohydroxyacetophenone

1. 2-Bromo-4′-Hydroxyacetophenone, 1-(4-Hydroxyphenyl)-2-Bromoethanone

CAS Registry Number [2491–38–5]

2. 2-Bromo-2′-Hydroxyacetophenone, (6CI, 7CI, 8CI)

CAS Registry Number [2491–36–3]

3. 5′-Bromo-2′-Hydroxy-Acetophenone (6CI, 7CI, 8CI), 1-(5-Bromo-2-Hydroxyphenyl)Ethanone

CAS Registry Number [1450–75–5]

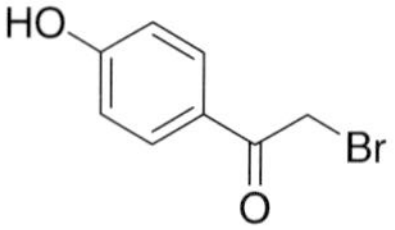

1.

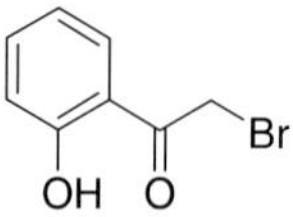

2.

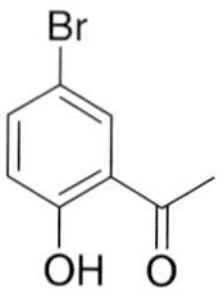

3.

Those substances are biocides used in emulsions, paints, adhesives, waxes, and polishes. They are both irritants and sensitizers. 2-Bromo-4'-hydroxyacetophenone used as a slimicide provoked sensitization after an accidental spillage, and recurrent allergic contact dermatitis at a workplace.

Suggested Reading
Jensen CD, Andersen KE (2003) Allergic contact dermatitis from a paper mill slimicide containing 2-bromo-4'-hydroxyacetophenone. Am J Contact Dermat 14:41–43

65. Bronopol

2-Bromo 2-Nitro 1,3-Propanediol

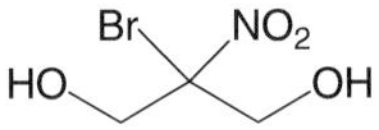

CAS Registry Number [52–51–7]

Bronopol is a preservative sometimes considered as a formaldehyde releaser. It was reported to be an allergen in cosmetics, cleaning agents, in dairy workers, and in a lubricant jelly used for ultrasound examination.

Suggested Reading
Grattan CEH, Harman RRM, Tan RSH (1986) Milk recorder dermatitis. Contact Dermatitis 14:217–220
Wilson CL, Powell SM (1990) An unusual cause of allergic contact dermatitis in a veterinary surgeon. Contact Dermatitis 23:42–43

66. Budesonide

Budesonide

CAS Registry number [51333–22–3]

R-Budesonide

CAS Registry Number [51372–29–3]

S-Budesonide

CAS Registry Number [51372–28–2]

R-Budesonide

S-Budesonide

Budesonide is a corticosteroid, a blend of two diastereosiomers.

R-Budesonide is a marker of the B group of corticosteroids. Such molecules have a *cis*-diol moiety or an acetal moiety on the C_{16} and C_{17} of the D cycle. One side chain is possible on C_{21}. The B group comprises amcinonide, budesonide, desonide or prednacinolone, flunisolide, fluocinolone and its acetonide, fluocinonide, fluclorolone and its acetonide, halcinonide, and acetonide, benetonide, diacetate and hexacetonide of triamcinolone.

S-Budesonide is a marker of the D2 group of corticosteroids. Such molecules are nonmethylated in C_{16} and have an ester function in C_{17}. They comprise hydrocortisone 17-butyrate, hydrocortisone-17-valerate, hydrocortisone aceponate, methylprednisolone aceponate, and prednicarbate.

Suggested Reading

Lepoittevin JP, Drieghe J, Dooms-Goossens A (1995) Studies in patients with corticosteroid contact allergy. Understanding cross-reactivity among different steroids. Arch Dermatol 131:31–37

Le Coz CJ (2002) Fiche d'éviction en cas d'hypersensibilité aux corticoïdes. Ann Dermatol Venereol 129:346–347

Le Coz CJ (2002) Fiche d'éviction en cas d'hypersensibilité au 17 butyrate d'hydrocortisone. Ann Dermatol Venereol 129:931

Le Coz CJ (2002) Fiche d'éviction en cas d'hypersensibilité au budésonide. Ann Dermatol Venereol 129:1409–1410

67. 1,4-Butanediol Diglycidyl Ether

CAS Registry Number
[2425–79–8]

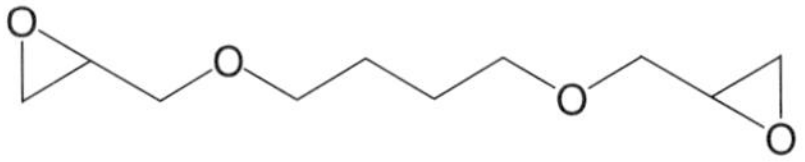

This substance is a reactive diluent in epoxy resins.

Suggested Reading

Jolanki R, Estlander T, Kanerva L (1987) Contact allergy to an epoxy reactive diluent: 1,4-butanediol diglycidyl ether. Contact Dermatitis 16: 87–92

Jolanki R, Kanerva L, Estlander T, Tarvainen K, Keskinen H, Henriks-Eckerman ML (1990) Occupational dermatoses from epoxy resin compounds. Contact Dermatitis 23:172–183

68. *N-tert*-Butyl-bis-(2-Benzothiazole) Sulfenamide

CAS Registry Number
[3741–80–8]

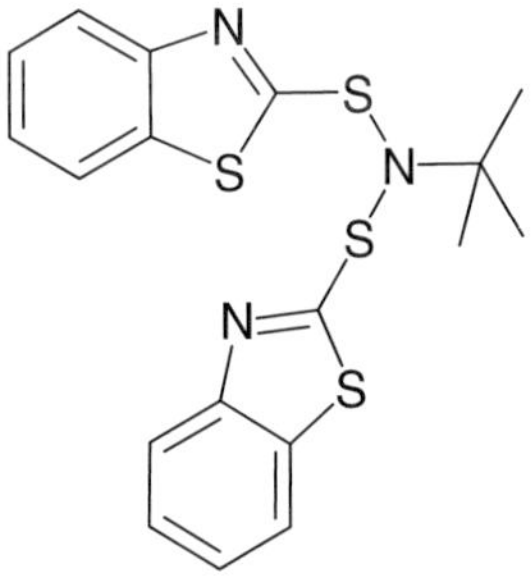

This mercaptobenzothiazole-sulfenamide chemical is used as an accelerator in rubber vulcanization.

Suggested Reading

Le Coz CJ (2004) Fiche d'éviction en cas d'hypersensibilité au mercapto-benzothiazole et au mercapto mix. Ann Dermatol Venereol 131: 846–848

69. Butyl Carbitol

Diethylene Glycol Monobutyl Ether

CAS Registry Number [112–34–5]

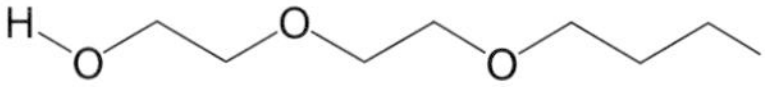

This organic solvent belongs to the carbitols group, and is included in waterbased liquids such as paints, surface cleaners, polishes and disinfectants. It is considered to be an exceptional allergen.

Suggested Reading

Berlin K, Johanson G, Lindberg M (1995) Hypersensitivity to 2-(2-butoxyethoxy)ethanol. Contact Dermatitis 32:54

Schliemann-Willers S, Bauer A, Elsner P (2000) Occupational contact dermatitis from diethylene glycol monobutyl ether in a podiatrist. Contact Dermatitis 43:225

70. *p-tert*-Butyl Catechol

CAS Registry Number [98–29–3]

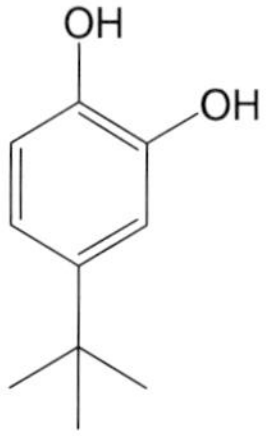

para-tert-Butyl catechol is specially prepared by reacting the impure catechol fraction with tertiary butyl alcohol. It is used for its various properties (inhibitor of polymerization and antioxidizing agent) in the manufacture of rubber, plastics and paints, in the preparation of petrolatum products, and as an anti-oxidant in oils. It may induce vitiligo.

Suggested Reading

Gawkrodger DJ, Cork MJ, Bleehen SS (1991) Occupational vitiligo and contact sensitivity to para-tertiary butyl catechol. Contact Dermatitis 25:200–201

71. *n*-Butyl Glycidyl Ether

CAS Registry Number [2426–08–6]

A reactive diluent used to reduce viscosity of epoxy resins Bisphenol A type.

Suggested Reading

Holness DL, Nethercott JR (1993) The performance of specialized collections of bisphenol A epoxy resin system components in the evaluation of workers in an occupational health clinic population. Contact Dermatitis 28 : 216–219

Jolanki R, Kanerva L, Estlander T, Tarvainen K, Keskinen H, Henriks-Eckerman ML (1990) Occupational dermatoses from epoxy resin compounds. Contact Dermatitis 23 : 172–183

72. *tert*-Butyl-Hydroquinone

2-*tert*-Butylhydroquinone, TBHQ

CAS Registry Number [1948–33–0]

This antioxidant has seldom been reported as a sensitizer, mainly in cosmetics (lipsticks, lip-gloss, hair dyes) or in cutting oils. Simultaneous/cross-reactions have been described to butylhydroxyanisole (BHA) and less frequently to butylhydroxytoluene (BHT) but not to hydroquinone.

Suggested Reading

Aalto-Korte K (2000) Allergic contact dermatitis from tertiary-butyl-hydroquinone (TBHQ) in a vegetable hydraulic oil. Contact Dermatitis 43 : 303

Le Coz CJ, Schneider GA (1998) Contact dermatitis from tertiary-butyl-hydroquinone in a hair dye, with cross-sensitivity to BHA and BHT. Contact Dermatitis 39 : 39–40

73. *p-tert*-Butyl-alpha-Methylhydrocinnamic Aldehyde

Lilial®, 2-(4-*tert*-Butylbenzyl)Propionaldehyde,
4-(1,1-Dimethylethyl)-α-Methyl-Benzenepropanal,
***p-tert*-Butyl-α-Methylhydrocinnamaldehyde, Lilestral**

CAS Registry Number [80–54–6]

Lilial® is a synthetic compound listed as a fragrance allergen. Its presence is indicated on cosmetics within the EU.

Suggested Reading

Giménez-Arnau E, Andersen KE, Bruze M, Frosch PJ, Johansen JD, Menné T, Rastogi SC, White IR, Lepoittevin JP (2000) Identification of Lilial as a fragrance sensitizer in a perfume by bioassay-guided chemical fractionation and structure-activity relationships. Contact Dermatitis 43: 351–358

74. Butylene Glycol

1,3-Butylene Glycol, 1,3-Butanediol

CAS Registry Number [107–88–0]

This dihydric alcohol is used for its humectant and preservative potentiator properties in cosmetics, topical medicaments and polyurethane, polyester, cellophane, and cigarettes. It has similar properties but is less irritant than propylene glycol. Contact allergies seem to be rare.

Suggested Reading

Diegenant C, Constandt L, Goossens A (2000) Allergic contact dermatitis due to 1,3-butylene glycol. Contact Dermatitis 43:324–235

Matsunaga K, Sugai T, Katoh J, Hayakawa R, Kozuka T, Itoh J, Tsuyuki S, Hosono K (1997) Group study on contact sensitivity of 1,3-butylene glycol. Environ Dermatol 4:195–205

75. *Para-tert*-Butylphenol

CAS Registry Number [98–54–4]

Para-tert-butylphenol is used with formaldehyde to produce the polycondensate *p-tert*-butylphenol formaldehyde resins (PTBPFR). Major occupational sources are neoprene glues and adhesives in industry, in the shoemaking and leather industries or in car production. It is also used as a box preservative in box and furniture manufacture, and in the production of casting molds, car brake linings, insulated electrical cables, adhesives, printing inks, and paper laminates. *Para-tert*-butyl-phenol seems to be the sensitizer.

Suggested Reading

Handley J, Todd D, Bingham A, Corbett R, Burrows D (1993) Allergic contact dermatitis from *para-tertiary*-butylphenol-formaldehyde resin (PTBP-F-R) in Northern Ireland. Contact Dermatitis 29:144–146

Mancuso G, Reggiani M, Berdondini RM (1996) Occupational dermatitis in shoemakers. Contact Dermatitis 34:17–22

Shono M, Ezoe K, Kaniwa MA, Ikarashi Y, Kohma S, Nakamura A (1991) Allergic contact dermatitis from para-tertiary-butylphenol-formaldehyde resin (PTBP-FR) in athletic tape and leather adhesive. Contact Dermatitis 24:281–288

Tarvainen K (1995) Analysis of patients with allergic patch test reactions to a plastics and glue series. Contact Dermatitis 32:346–351

76. Caffeic Acid Dimethyl Allylic Ester

3-Methyl-2-Butenyl-Caffeate

CAS Registry Number [108084–13–7]

This is the major allergen of poplar bud resins and of propolis, the bee glue derived almost exclusively from poplar buds.

Suggested Reading

Lamminpää A, Estlander T, Jolanki R, Kanerva L (1996) Occupational allergic contact dermatitis caused by decorative plants. Contact Dermatitis 34:330–335

Oliwiecki S, Beck MH, Hausen BM (1992) Occupational contact dermatitis from caffeates in poplar bud resin in a tree surgeon. Contact Dermatitis 27:127–128

77. Captafol

CAS Registry Number
[2425-06-1]

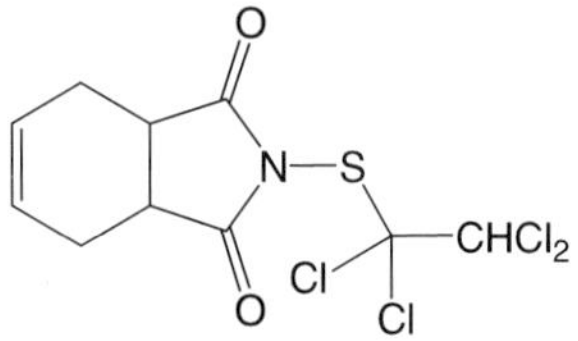

Captafol is a pesticide, belonging to thiophthalimide group. Occupational contact dermatitis was reported in an agricultural worker who had multiple sensitizations.

Suggested Reading

Peluso AM, Tardio M, Adamo F, Venturo N (1991) Multiple sensitization due to bis-dithiocarbamate and thiophthalimide pesticides. Contact Dermatitis 25:327

78. Captan

Captane, N-Trichloromethylmercaptotetrahydrophtalimide

CAS Registry Number
[133-06-2]

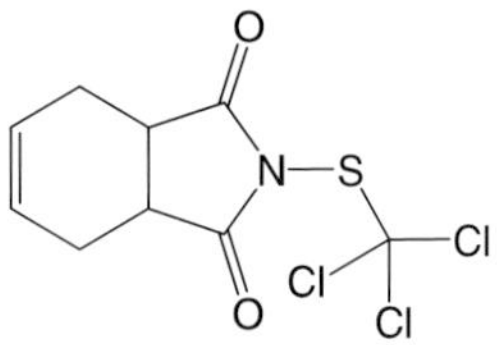

A pesticide, belonging to the thiophthalimide group, mainly affecting agricultural workers. Sensitizer and photosensitizer, it can induce contact urticaria. It is used as a fungicide and a bacteriostatic agent in cosmetics and toiletries, particularly in shampoos. Cases of contact dermatitis were reported in painters, polishers, and varnishers.

Suggested Reading

Aguirre A, Manzano D, Zabala R, Raton JA, Diaz-Perez JL (1994) Contact allergy to captan in a hairdresser. Contact Dermatitis 31:46

Moura C, Dias M, Vale T (1994) Contact dermatitis in painters, polishers and varnishers. Contact Dermatitis 31:51–53

O'Malley M, Rodriguez P, Maibach HI (1995) Pesticide patch testing: California nursery workers and controls. Contact Dermatitis 32:61–62

Peluso AM, Tardio M, Adamo F, Venturo N (1991) Multiple sensitization due to bis-dithiocarbamate and thiophthalimide pesticides. Contact Dermatitis 25:327

Vilaplana J, Romaguera C (1993) Captan, a rare contact sensitizer in hairdressing. Contact Dermatitis 29:107

79. Carbaryl

CAS Registry Number [63–25–2]

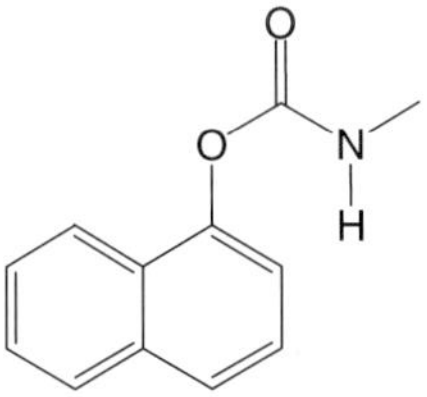

Carbaryl is a pesticide, insecticide, of the carbonate group. It induced sensitization in a farmer.

Suggested Reading

Sharma VK, Kaur S (1990) Contact sensitization by pesticides in farmers. Contact Dermatitis 23:77–80

80. Carbodiimide

Cyanamide

CAS Registry Number [420–04–2]

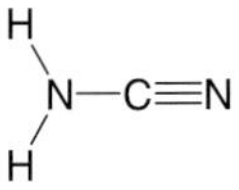

Cyanamide and its salts are used in various occasions such as in chemistry, in anti-rust solutions or in a drug (Come®) for treating alcoholism.

Suggested Reading
Goday Bujan JJ, Yanguas Bayona I, Arechavala RS (1994) Allergic contact dermatitis from cyanamide: report of 3 cases. Contact Dermatitis 31: 331–332

81. Carbofuran

CAS Registry Number [1563–66–2]

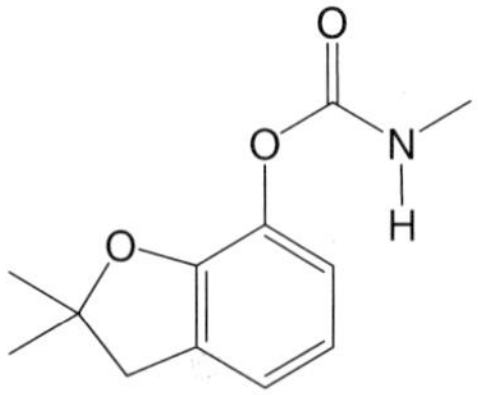

It is a pesticide with insecticide properties, of the carbamate group. It was implicated as a sensitizer in two farmers.

Suggested Reading
Sharma VK, Kaur S (1990) Contact sensitization by pesticides in farmers. Contact Dermatitis 23:77–80

82. Cardols

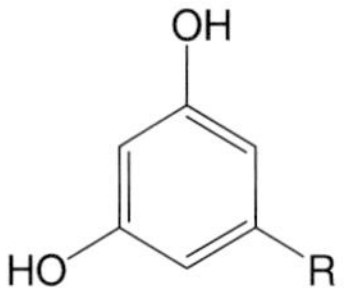

Cardols are a mixture of several analog molecules with an alkyl chain (-R) with 13, 15, 17, or 19 carbon and 0–3 unsaturations. One of the main cashew nut shell liquid components, along with anacardic acid. Sensitization occurs in cashew nut workers.

Suggested Reading
Diogenes MJN, De Morais SM, Carvalho FF (1996) Contact dermatitis among cashew nut workers. Contact Dermatitis 35:114–115

83. Δ-3-Carene

CAS Registry Number
[13466–78–9]

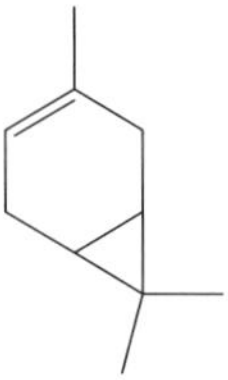

Hydroperoxides of Δ-3-carene are allergens contained in turpentine. Occupational exposure occurs in painters, varnishers, or in ceramic decoration. The percentage of Δ-3-carene is higher in Indonesian than in Portuguese turpentine.

Suggested Reading
Lear JT, Heagerty AHM, Tan BB, Smith AG, English JSC (1996) Transient re-emergence of oil turpentine allergy in the pottery industry. Contact Dermatitis 35:169–172

84. Carteolol

CAS Registry Number
[51781–06–7]

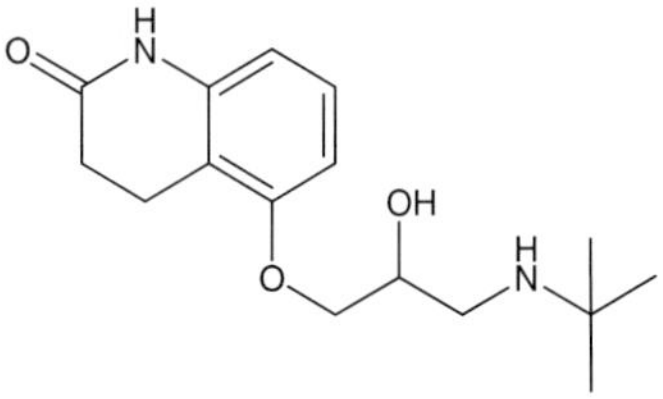

Carteolol was implicated in allergic contact dermatitis due to beta-blockers agents in eye-drops.

Suggested Reading
Giordano-Labadie F, Lepoittevin JP, Calix I, Bazex J (1997) Allergie de contact aux â-bloqueurs des collyres: allergie croisée? Ann Dermatol Venereol 124:322–324

85. CD1

N,N-Diethylparaphenylenediamine Monochlorhydrate

CAS Registry Number [2198–58–5]

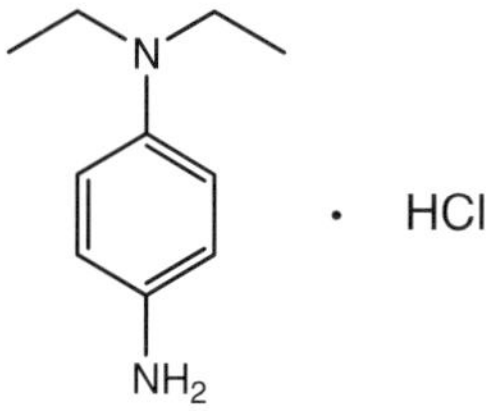

A color film developer. It is an allergen and an irritant in photographers. Cross-reactivity is possible with Disperse Blue 124, Disperse Blue 106, and Disperse red 17 but not with *para*-amino compounds.

Suggested Reading

Aguirre A, Landa N, Gonzalez M, Diaz-Perez JL (1992) Allergic contact dermatitis in a photographer. Contact Dermatitis 27:340–341

Galindo PA, Garcia R, Garrido JA, Feo F, Fernandez F (1994) Allergic contact dermatitis from colour developers: absence of cross-sensitivity to para-amino compounds. Contact Dermatitis 30:301

Hansson C, Ahlfors S, Bergendorff O (1997) Concomitant contact dermatitis due to textile dyes and to colour film developers can be explained by the formation of the same hapten. Contact Dermatitis 37:27–31

Lidén C, Brehmer-Andersson E (1988) Occupational dermatoses from colour developing agents. Clinical and histopathological observations. Acta Derm Venereol (Stockh) 68:514–522

86. CD2

4-*N,N*-Diethyl-2-Methyl-1,4-Phenylenediamine (Hydrochloride)

CAS Registry Number [2051–79–8]

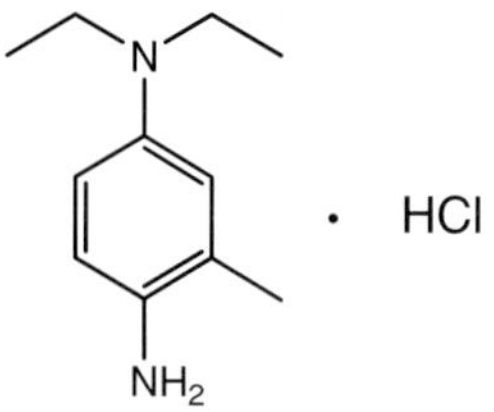

A color film developer. It acts as an allergen and an irritant in photographers. Cross-reactivity is possible with Disperse Blue 124, Disperse Blue 106, and Disperse Red 17 but not to *para*-amino compounds.

Suggested Reading

Aguirre A, Landa N, Gonzalez M, Diaz-Perez JL (1992) Allergic contact dermatitis in a photographer. Contact Dermatitis 27:340–341

Galindo PA, Garcia R, Garrido JA, Feo F, Fernandez F (1994) Allergic contact dermatitis from colour developers: absence of cross-sensitivity to para-amino compounds. Contact Dermatitis 30:301

Hansson C, Ahlfors S, Bergendorff O (1997) Concomitant contact dermatitis due to textile dyes and to colour film developers can be explained by the formation of the same hapten. Contact Dermatitis 37:27–31

Lidén C, Brehmer-Andersson E (1988) Occupational dermatoses from colour developing agents. Clinical and histopathological observations. Acta Derm Venereol (Stockh) 68:514–522

Rustemeyer T, Frosch PJ (1995) Allergic contact dermatitis from colour film developers. Contact Dermatitis 32:59–60

87. CD3

4-(Ethyl-*N*-2-Methan-Sulfonamidoethyl)-2-Methyl-1,4-Phenylenediamine (*1,5H$_2$SO$_4$ *H$_2$O)

CAS Registry Number
[25646–71–3]

$\cdot \quad H_2SO_4$

A color film developer. It caused some allergic reactions in photographers. Cross-reactivity is possible with Disperse Blue 124, Disperse Blue 106, and Disperse Red 17

Suggested Reading

Aguirre A, Landa N, Gonzalez M, Diaz-Perez JL (1992) Allergic contact dermatitis in a photographer. Contact Dermatitis 27:340–341

Galindo PA, Garcia R, Garrido JA, Feo F, Fernandez F (1994) Allergic contact dermatitis from colour developers: absence of cross-sensitivity to para-amino compounds. Contact Dermatitis 30:301

Hansson C, Ahlfors S, Bergendorff O (1997) Concomitant contact dermatitis due to textile dyes and to colour film developers can be explained by the formation of the same hapten. Contact Dermatitis 37:27–31

Lidén C, Brehmer-Andersson E (1988) Occupational dermatoses from colour developing agents. Clinical and histopathological observations. Acta Derm Venereol (Stockh) 68:514–522

Rustemeyer T, Frosch PJ (1995) Allergic contact dermatitis from colour developers. Contact Dermatitis 32:59–60

Scheman AJ, Katta R (1997) Photographic allergens: an update. Contact Dermatitis 37:130

88. CD4

4-(Ethyl-*N*-Hydroxyethyl)-2-Methyl-1,4-Phenylenediamine (*H_2SO_4*H_2O)

CAS Registry Number
[25646–77–9]

$\cdot$ H_2SO_4

Color film developer. It is both an allergen and an irritant in photographers. Cross-reactivity is possible with Disperse Blue 124, Disperse Blue 106, and Disperse Red 17.

Suggested Reading

Aguirre A, Landa N, Gonzalez M, Diaz-Perez JL (1992) Allergic contact dermatitis in a photographer. Contact Dermatitis 27:340–341

Galindo PA, Garcia R, Garrido JA, Feo F, Fernandez F (1994) Allergic contact dermatitis from colour developers: absence of cross-sensitivity to para-amino compounds. Contact Dermatitis 30:301

Hansson C, Ahlfors S, Bergendorff O (1997) Concomitant contact dermatitis due to textile dyes and to colour film developers can be explained by the formation of the same hapten. Contact Dermatitis 37:27–31

Lidén C, Brehmer-Andersson E (1988) Occupational dermatoses from colour developing agents. Clinical and histopathological observations. Acta Derm Venereol (Stockh) 68:514–522

Rustemeyer T, Frosch PJ (1995) Allergic contact dermatitis from colour developers. Contact Dermatitis 32:59–60

Scheman AJ, Katta R (1997) Photographic allergens: an update. Contact Dermatitis 37:130

89. CD6

4-Amino-*N*-Ethyl-*N*-(2-Methoxyethyl)-2-Methyl Paraphenylenediamine di-*p*-Toluene Sulfonate

CAS Registry Number [50928–80–8]

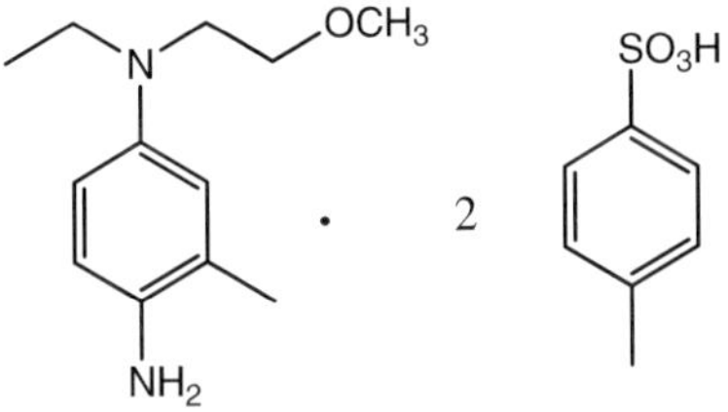

This color film developer rarely induced contact dermatitis in photographers.

Suggested Reading

Lidén C (1989) Occupational dermatoses at a film laboratory. Contact Dermatitis 20:191–200

Lidén C, Brehmer-Andersson E (1988) Occupational dermatoses from colour developing agents. Clinical and histopathological observations. Acta Derm Venereol (Stockh) 68:514–522

90. Cefaclor

CAS Registry Number [70356–03–5]

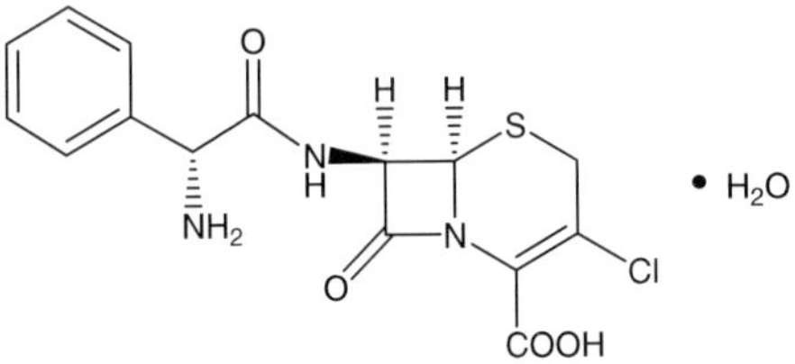

Cefaclor is a semi-synthetic cephalosporin antibiotic, related to cefalexin, and a frequent inducer of serum sickness-like reactions.

Suggested Reading

Hebert AA, Sigman ES, Levy ML (1991) Serum sickness-like reactions from cefaclor in children. J Am Acad Dermatol 25:805–808

91. Cephalosporins

R^1 with structure showing cephem nucleus:

$$R^1 - C(=O) - N(H) - \text{(cephem nucleus with S, N, COOH)} - R^2$$

All cephalosporins have a 7-amino-cephalosporanic group (cephem nucleus). They differ by a C$_7$ and a C$_3$ substitution. The cause of an allergic reaction to cephalosporins can be the cephem nucleus itself, but this seems to be rare. Allergic contact dermatitis from cephalosporins is uncommon and mainly occurs in health-care, pharmaceutical, and veterinary professions. Systemic drug reactions are more frequent, and can involve an immuno-allergic mechanism or not. Some of them are severe and life threatening.

Cefaclor is frequently responsible for serum thickness diseases. Cefotaxime, ceftizoxime, ceftazidime, ceftriaxone and cefodizime, several third-generation cephalosporins, caused positive patch reactions in a sensitized nurse. Cefazoline, cefoxitin, ceftriaxone, and ceftazidime were responsible for contact dermatitis in a nurse. Sensitivity to cephalothin, cephamandol and cephazolin, cephalosporins of the first and second generation, was reported in a pharmaceutical laboratory analyst. Ceftiofur sodium, a third-generation veterinary cephalosporin, caused contact dermatitis in two chicken vaccinators. No cross-sensitivity was observed to other cephalosporins. Cephalexin hypersensitivity was reported in three cases, and to cefuroxime in one case with cross-reaction to cephalotin and cephaloridine.

Suggested Reading
Condé-Salazar L, Guimaraens D, Romero LV, Gonzales MA (1986) Occupational dermatitis from cephalosporins. Contact Dermatitis 14:70–71
Filipe P, Soares Almeida RSL, Guerra Rodrigo F (1996) Occupational allergic contact dermatitis from cephalosporins. Contact Dermatitis 34:226
Foti C, Vena GA, Cucurachi MR, Angelini G (1994) Occupational contact allergy from cephalosporins. Contact Dermatitis 31:129–130
Garcia-Bravo B, Gines E, Russo F (1995) Occupational contact dermatitis from ceftiofur sodium. Contact Dermatitis 33:62–63
Romano A, Pietrantonio F, Di Fonso M, Venuti A (1992) Delayed hypersensitivity to cefuroxime. Contact Dermatitis 27:270–271

92. Cetearyl Isononanoate

Cetearyl Hexadecyl Isononanoate

CAS Registry Number [84878–33–1]

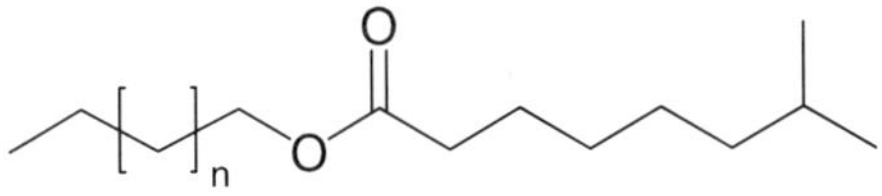

n: 14 to 16

This substance results from esterification of a saturated C_{16} to C_{18} alcohol, namely cetyl or stearyl alcohol, and a branched chain isononanoic acid. It is used as a hair conditioning agent, a skin conditioning agent, and an emollient, and is found in several moisturizing creams.

Suggested Reading

Le Coz CJ, Bressieux A (2003) Allergic contact dermatitis from cetearyl isononanoate. Contact Dermatitis 48:343

93. Chloramphenicol

CAS Registry Number [56–75–7]

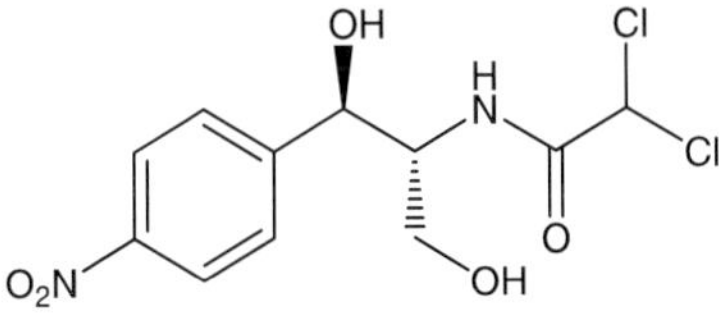

This broad spectrum phenicol group antibiotic has been implicated in allergic contact dermatitis. Cross-sensitivity to thiamphenicol is possible but not systematic.

Suggested Reading

Le Coz CJ, Santinelli F (1998) Facial contact dermatitis from chloramphenicol with cross-sensitivity to thiamphenicol. Contact Dermatitis 38:108–109

94. Chlorhexidine (Digluconate)

CAS Registry Number [55–56–1] (CAS Registry Number [18472–51–0])

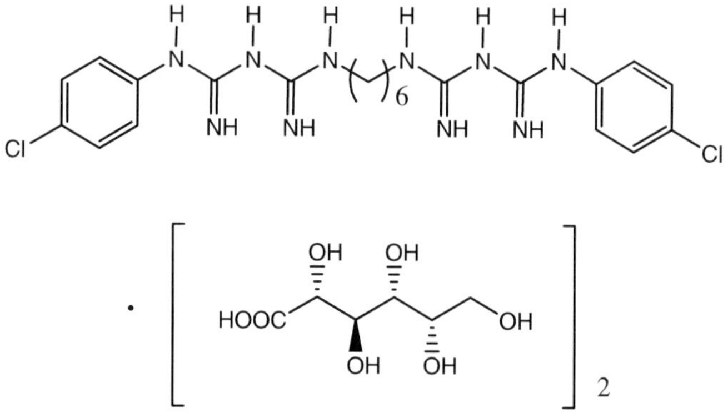

Chlorhexidine is a broad-spectrum antimicrobial agent, a synthetic biguanide antiseptic and disinfectant, available under different forms (diacetate, dihydrochloride, and mostly digluconate). It is also used as a biocide in several topicals and cosmetics. It may cause allergic contact dermatitis, photosensitivity or even fixed drug eruption, mainly after prolonged and repeated applications in health workers, leg ulcer, and leg eczema patients. Immediate-type reactions have been reported: contact urticaria, asthma, and anaphylactic shock.

Suggested Reading

Krautheim AB, Jermann THM, Bircher AJ (2004) Chlorhexidine anaphyl-axis: case report and review of the literature. Contact Dermatitis 50: 113–116

Rudzki E, Rebandel P, Grzywa Z (1989) Patch tests with occupational contactants in nurses, doctors and dentists. Contact Dermatitis 20: 247–250

95. 5-Chloro-1-Methyl-4-Nitroimidazole

CAS Registry Number [4897–25–0]

This intermediate in azathioprine synthesis is also present in the end product. It induced contact dermatitis in a man working on azathioprine synthesis. Cross-reactivity is possible with imidazoles tioconazole and econazole.

Suggested Reading

Jolanki R, Alanko K, Pfäffli P, Estlander T, Kanerva L (1997) Occupational allergic contact dermatitis from 5-chloro-1-methyl-4-nitroimidazole. Contact Dermatitis 36:53–54

96. Chloroacetamide

CAS Registry Number [79–07–2]

Chloroacetamide is as a preservative used in several applications as in cutting metalworking fluids, in paints or in glues. It can induce contact dermatitis in hairdressers or in shoemakers, being used as a leather preservative.

Suggested Reading

Katsarou A, Koufou B, Takou K, Kalogeromitros D, Papanayiotou G, Vareltzidis A (1995) Patch test results in hairdressers with contact dermatitis in Greece (1985–1994). Contact Dermatitis 33:347–348
Mancuso G, Reggiani M, Berdondini RM (1996) Occupational dermatitis in shoemakers. Contact Dermatitis 34:17–22

97. Chloroacetophenone

CAS Registry Number [532–27–4]

ω-Chloroacetophenone is contained in tear gases (lacrimators). This substance has important irritative potential but can also be a sensitizer.

Suggested Reading

Brand CU, Schmidli J, Ballmer-Weber B, Hunziker T (1995) Lymphozyten-stimulationstest, eine mögliche Alternative zur Sicherung einer Cloracetophenon-Sensibilisierung. Hautarzt 46:702–704

98. Chloroatranol

CAS Registry Number [57074–21–2]

Chloroatranol has recently been identified as a constituent and major allergen in oak moss absolute, a frequent allergen in people sensitized to perfumes. This potent allergen gives reactions with concentrations down to 5 ppm in sensitized patients. It may cross-react with atranol.

Suggested Reading

Bernard G, Giménez-Arnau E, Rastogi SC et al (2003) Contact allergy to oak moss: search for sensitizing molecules using combined bioassay-guided chemical fractionation, GC-MS and structure-activity relation-ship analysis (part 1). Arch Dermatol Res 295:229–235

Johansen JD, Andersen KE, Svedman C, Bruze M, Bernard G, Giménez-Arnau E, Rastogi SC, Lepoittevin JP, Menné T (2003) Chloroatranol, an extremely potent allergen hidden in perfumes: a dose response elicita-tion study. Contact Dermatitis 49:180–184

99. Chlorocresol

4-Chloro-3-methylphenol, Parachlorometacresol, 2-Chloro-5-hydroxytoluene

CAS Registry Number [59–50–7]

Chlorocresol is a biocide used for its disinfectant and preservative properties, in topicals or in cutting fluid.

Suggested Reading

Le Coz CJ, Scrivener Y, Santinelli F, Heid E (1998) Sensibilisation de contact au cours des ulcères de jambe. Ann Dermatol Venereol 125: 694–699

Walker SL, Chalmers RJ, Beck MH (2004) Contact urticaria due to p-chlorom-cresol. Br J Dermatol 151:936–937

100. Chlorophorin

CAS Registry Number [537–41–7]

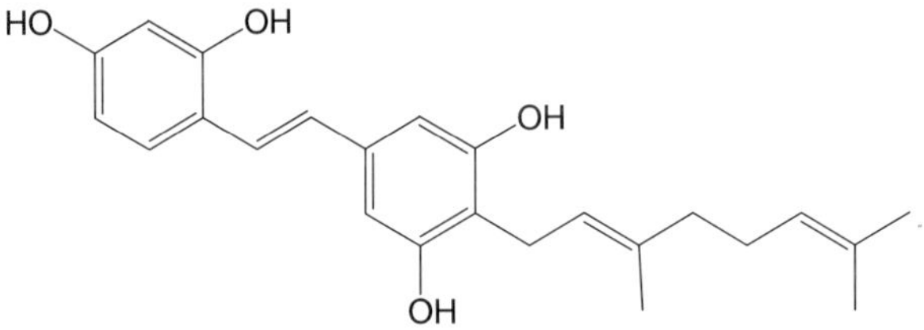

Chlorophorin is the allergen in iroko, kambala (*Chlorophora excelsa*). Occupational dermatitis can occurs in woodworkers.

Suggested Reading

Lamminpää A, Estlander T, Jolanki R, Kanerva L (1996) Occupational allergic contact dermatitis caused by decorative plants. Contact Dermatitis 34:330–335

101. Chlorothalonil

2,4,5,6–1,3-Tetrachloroisophtalonitrile, 1,3-Dicyano Tetrachlorobenzene, Daconil®

CAS Registry Number [1897–45–6]

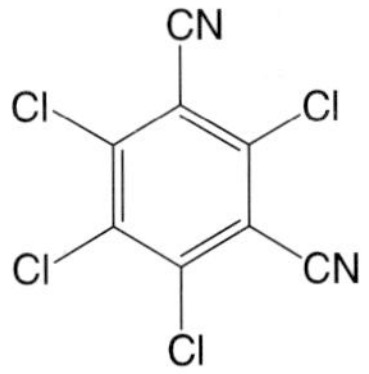

Chlorothalonil is a fungicide widely used in the cultivation of or-
namental plants and flowers, rice, and onions. In banana planta-
tions it is used in fumigations by airplanes. It can be used as a
preservative of paints and of woods. It can induce contact
urticaria, irritant and allergic contact dermatitis, erythema dyschromicum perstans or folliculitis mainly in agricultural workers,
wood-related professions or in horticulturists.

Suggested Reading

Boman A, Montelius J, Rissanen RL, Lidén C (2000) Sensitizing potential
of chlorothalonil in the guinea pig and the mouse. Contact Dermatitis
43:273–279
Meding B (1986) Contact dermatitis from tetrachloroisophtalonitrile in
paint. Contact Dermatitis 15:187
O'Malley M, Rodriguez P, Maibach HI (1995) Pesticide patch testing: California nursery workers and controls. Contact Dermatitis 32:61–62
Penagos H, Jimenez V, Fallas V, O'Malley M, Maibach HI (1996) Chlorothalonil, a possible cause of erythema dyschromicum perstants (ashy
dermatitis). Contact Dermatitis 35:214–218

102. Chlorpromazine

CAS Registry Number [50–53–3]

This phenothiazine with sedative properties is used in human
medicine and induced contact dermatitis in nurses or those working in the pharmaceutical industry. It is also in veterinary medicine, to avoid mortality of pigs during transportation. It is a sensitizer and a photosensitizer.

Suggested Reading

Brasch J, Hessler HJ, Christophers E (1991) Occupational (photo)allergic
contact dermatitis from azaperone in a piglet dealer. Contact Dermatitis 25:258–259

103. Cinnamal

Cinnamic Aldehyde, Cinnamaldehyde, 3-Phenyl-2-Propenal

CAS Registry Number [104–55–2]

This perfumed molecule is used as a fragrance in perfumes, a flavoring agent in soft drinks, ice creams, dentifrices, pastries, chewing-gum, etc. It can induce both contact urticaria and delayed-type reactions. It can be responsible for dermatitis in the perfume industry or in food handlers. Cinnamic aldehyde is contained in "fragrance mix." As a fragrance allergen, it has to be mentioned by name in cosmetics within the EU.

Suggested Reading

Nethercott JR, Holness DL (1989) Occupational dermatitis in food handlers and bakers. J Am Acad Dermatol 21:485–490

Seite-Bellezza D, El Sayed F, Bazex J (1994) Contact urticaria from cinnamic aldehyde and benzaldehyde in a confectioner. Contact Dermatitis 31:272–273

104. Cinnamyl Alcohol

Cinnamic Alcohol, 3-Phenyl-2-Propenol

CAS Registry Number [104–54–1]

Cinnamyl alcohol occurs (in esterified form) in storax, *Myroxylon pereirae*, cinnamon leaves, and hyacinth oil. It is obtained by the alkaline hydrolysis of storax, and prepared synthetically by reducing cinnamal diacetate with iron filings and acetic acid, and from cinnamaldehyde by Meerwein–Ponndorf reduction with aluminum isopropoxide. Cinnamic alcohol is contained in the "fragrance mix." As a fragrance allergen, it has to be mentioned by name in cosmetics within the EU. Occupational cases of contact dermatitis were reported in perfume industry. Patch tests can be positive in food handlers.

Suggested Reading

Gutman SG, Somov BA (1968) Allergic reactions caused by components of perfumery preparations. Vestn Dermatol Venereol 12:62–66

Nethercott JR, Holness DL (1989) Occupational dermatitis in food handlers and bakers. J Am Acad Dermatol 21:485–490

105. Citral

3,7-Dimethyl-2,6-Octadien-1-al,
Blend of Neral and Geranial,
Blend of (Z)-3,7-Dimethyl-2,6-Octadienal
and (E)-3,7-Dimethyl-2,6-Octadienal

CAS Registry Number [5392–40–5]
(CAS Registry Number [141–27–5] +
CAS Registry Number [106–26–3])

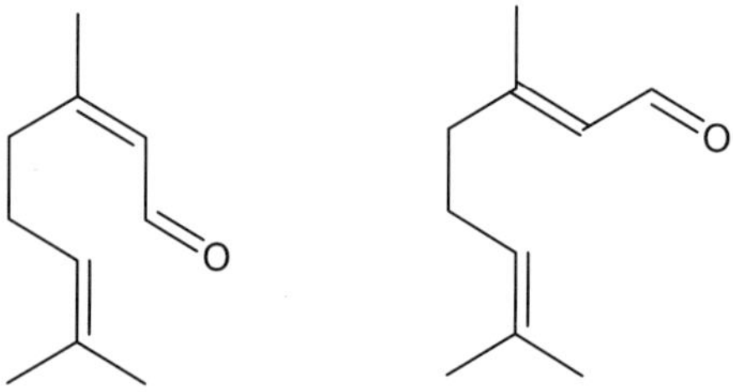

Neral   Geranial

Citral is an aldehyde fragrance and flavoring ingredient, a blend of isomers *cis* (Neral) and *trans* (geranial). As a fragrance allergen, citral has to be mentioned by name in cosmetics within the EU.

Suggested Reading

Frosch PJ, Johansen JD, Menné T, Pirker C, Rastogi SC, Andersen KE, Bruze M, Goossens A, Lepoittevin JP, White IR (2002) Further important sensitizers in patients sensitive to fragrances. Contact Dermatitis 47:78–85

106. Citronellol

3,7-Dimethyl-6-Octen-1-ol, Cephrol

CAS Registry Numbers [106–22–9] and [26489–01–0]

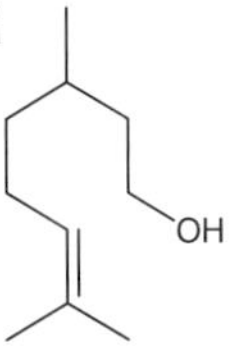

L-Citronellol is a constituent of rose and geranium oils. D-Citronellol occurs in Ceylon and Java citronella oils. As a fragrance allergen, citronellol has to be mentioned by name in cosmetics within the EU.

Suggested Reading

Frosch PJ, Johansen JD, Menné T, Pirker C, Rastogi SC, Andersen KE, Bruze M, Goossens A, Lepoittevin JP, White IR (2002) Further important sensitizers in patients sensitive to fragrances. Contact Dermatitis 47: 78–85

107. Clindamycin

Clindamycin

CAS Registry Number [18323–44–9]

Clindamycin Hydrochloride

CAS Registry Number [21462–39–5]

Clindamycin Phosphate

CAS Registry Number [24729–96–2]

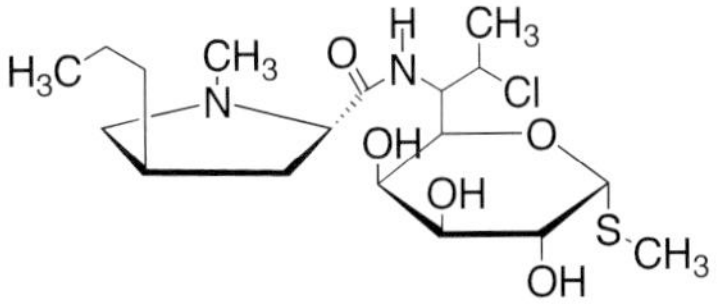

This lincosanide antibiotic is used in topical form for acne, or systemically has been responsible for exanthematous rashes and acute generalized exanthematous pustulosis.

Suggested Reading
Lammintausta K, Tokola R, Kalimo K (2002) Cutaneous adverse reactions to clindamycin: results of skin tests and oral exposure. Br J Dermatol 146:643–648
Valois M, Phillips EJ, Shear NH, Knowles SR (2003) Clindamycin-associated acute generalized exanthematous pustulosis. Contact Dermatitis 48:169

108. Clopidol

Methylchlorpindol, 3,5-Dichloro-2,6-Dimethyl-4-Pyridinol

CAS Registry Number [2971–90–6], [11116–46–4], [68821–99–8]

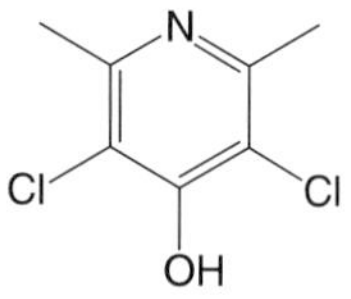

This drug is used for the prevention of coccidiosis in poultry.

Suggested Reading
Mancuso G, Staffa M, Errani A, Berdondini RM, Fabri P (1990) Occupational dermatitis in animal feed mill workers. Contact Dermatitis 22:37–41
Pang GF, Cao YZ, Fan CL, Zhang JJ, Li XM, MacNeil JD (2003) Determination of clopidol residues in chicken tissues by liquid chromatography: collaborative study. J AOAC Int 86:685–693

109. Cloxacillin

CAS Registry Number
[61–72–3]

Cloxacillin Sodium Monohydrate

CAS Registry Number:
[7081–44–9]

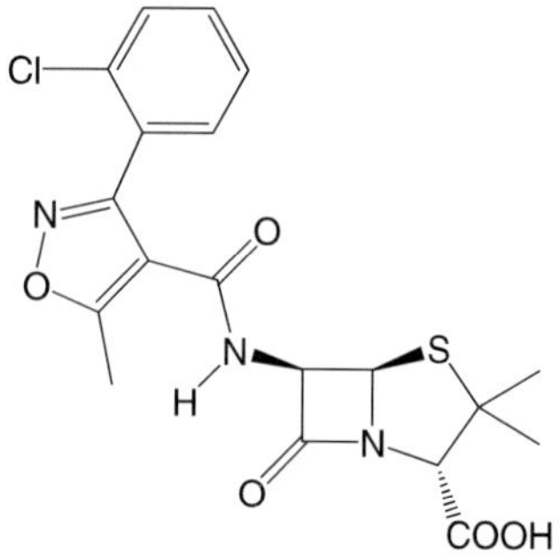

Cloxacillin is a semi-synthetic penicillin close to oxacillin. It induced contact dermatitis in a pharmaceutical factory worker with positive reactions to ampicillin but not to penicillin. In cutaneous drug reactions such as acute generalized exanthematous pustulosis due to amoxicillin, cross-reactivity is frequent to cloxacillin (personal observations).

Suggested Reading

Rudzki E, Rebandel P (1991) Hypersensitivity to semisynthetic penicillins but not to natural penicillin. Contact Dermatitis 25:192

110. Cobalt naphthenate

Naphthenic Acids, Cobalt Salts

CAS Registry Numbers [61789–51–3], [161279–65–8]

Cobalt naphthenate is made by treating cobalt hydroxide or acetate with naphthenic acid. It is an accelerant in rubber, unsaturated polyester, and vinyl ester resins.

Suggested Reading

Shena D, Rosina P, Chieregato C, Colombari R (1995) Lymphomatoid-like contact dermatitis from cobalt naphthenate. Contact Dermatitis 33: 197–198

Tarvainen K, Jolanki R, Forsman-Gronholm L, Estlander T, Pfaffli P, Juntunen J, Kanerva L (1993) Exposure, skin protection and occupational skin diseases in the glass-fibre-reinforced plastics industry. Contact Dermatitis 29:119–127

111. Cocamidopropyl Betaine

Cocoamphodipropionate, Cocamidopropyl Dimethyl Glycine, Cocoamphocarboxypropionate, Cocoyl Amide Propylbetaine, N-(2-Aminoethyl)-N-[2-(2-carboxyethoxy)ethyl] beta-Alanine

CAS Registry Numbers [61789–40–0], [83138–08–3], [86438–79–1]

Cocamidopropyl betaine is a pseudo-amphoteric zwitterion detergent derived from long-chain alkylbetaines. It is available from
many suppliers under more than 50 trade names (including Tego-
betain L7 and Ampholyt JB 130). Exposure occurs via rinse-off
products such as liquid soaps, shampoos, and shower gels, but
also via leave-on products (for example, roll-on deodorant). Occupational sources are mainly in hairdressing. The first synthesis
step consists of the reaction of coconut fatty acids with 3-dimethyl-
aminopropylamine, giving cocamidopropyl dimethylamine. This
amido-amine is converted into cocamidopropyl betaine by reaction with sodium monochloroacetate. Both dimethylaminopropylamine and cocamidopropyl dimethylamine are thought to be the
sensitizers.

Suggested Reading

Angelini G, Foti C, Rigano L, Vena GA (1995) 3-Dimethylaminopropyl-
    amine: a key substance in contact allergy to cocamidopropylbetaine?
    Contact Dermatitis 32 : 96–99
De Groot AC, van der Walle HB, Weyland JW (1995) Contact allergy to
    cocamidopropyl betaine. Contact Dermatitis 33 : 419–422
McFadden JP, Ross JS, White IR, Basketter DA (2001) Clinical allergy to
    cocamidopropyl betaine: reactivity to cocamidopropylamine and lack
    of reactivity to 3-dimethylaminopropylamine. Contact Dermatitis 45 :
    72–74

112. Cocamidopropyl Dimethylamine

N-[3-(Dimethylamino)Propyl]Coco Amides, 1-(N,N-Dimethylamino)-3-(Coconut Oil Amido)-Propane, Coconut Fatty Acid, Dimethylaminopropylamide

CAS Registry Number [68140–01–2]

This amido amine may be the allergen in cocamidopropyl betaine.

Suggested Reading

McFadden JP, Ross JS, White IR, Basketter DA (2001) Clinical allergy to cocamidopropyl betaine: reactivity to cocamidopropylamine and lack of reactivity to 3-dimethylaminopropylamine. Contact Dermatitis 45:72–74

113. Coconut Diethanolamide

Cocamide DEA, Coconut Oil Fatty Acids Diethanolamide,
N,N-bis(2-Hydroxyethyl)Coco Fatty Acid Diethanolamide,
Cocoyl Diethanolamide

CAS Registry Number [68603–42–9]

Cocamide DEA, manufactured from coconut oil, is widely used in industry and at home as a surface-active agent. It is contained in hand gels, hand washing soaps, shampoos, and dish-washing liquids for its foam-producing and stabilizing properties, and in metalworking fluids and polishing agents as an anticorrosion inhibitor.

Suggested Reading

Fowler JF Jr (1998) Allergy to cocamide DEA. Am J Contact Dermat 9:40–41

Kanerva L, Jolanki R, Estlander T (1993) Dentist's occupational allergic contact dermatitis caused by coconut diethanolamide, N-ethyl-4-toluene sulfonamide and 4-tolydietahnolamine. Acta Derm Venereol (Stockh) 73:126–129

Pinola A, Estlander T, Jolanki R, Tarvainen K, Kanerva L (1993) Occupational allergic contact dermatitis due to coconut diethanolamide (Cocamide DEA). Contact Dermatitis 29:262–265

114. Codeine (Phosphate, Hydrochloride)

Methylmorphine

CAS Registry Number [76–57–3]
(CAS Registry Number [52–28–8],
CAS Registry Number [1422–07–7])

Codeine has been reported as an occupational sensitizer in workers in the production of opium alkaloids. Codeine has been responsible for fixed drug eruptions or generalized dermatitis. Cross-sensitivity is expected to morphine.

Suggested Reading

Condé-Salazar L, Guimaraens D, Gonzalez M, Fuente C (1991) Occupational allergic contact dermatitis from opium alkaloids. Contact Dermatitis 25 : 202–203

Estrada JL, Alvarez Puebla MJ, Ortiz de Urbina JJ, Matilla B, Rodríguez Prieto MA, Gozalo F (2001) Generalized eczema due to codeine. Contact Dermatitis 44 : 185

Waclawski ER, Aldridge R (1995) Occupational dermatitis from thebaine and codeine. Contact Dermatitis 33 : 51

115. Costunolide

CAS Registry Number [553–21–9]

This germacranolide sesquiterpene lactone is extracted from costus oil. With alantolactone and dehydrocostunolide, it is a component of lactone mix used to elicit reactions in patients sensitive to Asteraceae–Compositae. An erythema-multiform-like occupational contact dermatitis case occurred in a chemical student after an accidental exposure to costus oil.

Suggested Reading

Ducombs G, Benezra C, Talaga P, Andersen KE, Burrows D, Camarasa JG, Dooms-Goossens A, Frosch PJ, Lachapelle JM, Menné T, Rycroft RJG, White IR, Shaw S, Wilkinson JD (1990) Patch testing with the "sesquiterpene lactone mix": a marker for contact allergy to Compositae and other sesquiterpene-lactone-containing plants. Contact Dermatitis 22 : 249–252

Le Coz CJ, Lepoittevin JP (2001) Occupational erythema-multiforme-like dermatitis from sensitization to costus resinoid, followed by flare-up and systemic contact dermatitis from beta-cyclocostunolide in a chemistry student. Contact Dermatitis 44 : 310–311

116. Coumarin

1-Benzopyran-2-one, *cis-o*-Coumarinic Acid Lactone

CAS Registry Number [91–64–5]

Coumarin is an aromatic lactone naturally occurring in Tonka beans and other plants. As a fragrance allergen, it has to be mentioned by name in cosmetics within the EU.

Suggested Reading

Frosch PJ, Johansen JD, Menné T, Pirker C, Rastogi SC, Andersen KE, Bruze M, Goossens A, Lepoittevin JP, White IR (2002) Further important sensitizers in patients sensitive to fragrances. Contact Dermatitis 47: 78–85

117. Cresyl Glycidyl Ether

CAS Registry Number [26447–14–3]

It is a reactive diluent added in epoxy resins Bisphenol A type.

Suggested Reading

Chieregato C, Vincenzi C, Guerra L, Farina P (1994) Occupational allergic contact dermatitis due to ethylenediamine dihydrochloride and cresyl glycidyl ether in epoxy resin systems. Contact Dermatitis 30: 120

Daecke C, Schaller J, Goos M (1994) Acrylates as potent allergens in occupational and domestic exposures. Contact Dermatitis 30: 190–191

Holness DL, Nethercott JR (1993) The performance of specialized collections of bisphenol A epoxy resin system components in the evaluation of workers in an occupational health clinic population. Contact Dermatitis 28: 216–219

Jolanki R, Kanerva L, Estlander T, Tarvainen K, Keskinen H, Henriks-Eckerman ML (1990) Occupational dermatoses from epoxy resin compounds. Contact Dermatitis 23: 172–183

118. Cyclohexanone

CAS Registry Number [108–94–1]

Used as a polyvinyl chloride solvent, cyclohexanone caused contact dermatitis in a woman manufacturing PVC fluidotherapy bags. Cyclohexanone probably does not cross-react with cyclohexanone resin. A cyclohexanone-derived resin used in paints and varnishes, caused contact dermatitis in painters.

Suggested Reading
Bruze M, Boman A, Bergquist-Karlson A, Björkner B, Wahlberg JE, Woog E (1988) Contact allergy to cyclohexanone resin in humans and guinea pigs. Contact Dermatitis 18 : 46–49
Sanmartin O, de la Cuadra J (1992) Occupational contact dermatitis from cyclohexanone as a PVC adhesive. Contact Dermatitis 27 : 189–190

119. 2-Cyclohexen-1-one

CAS Registry Number [930–68–7]

This strong sensitizer has been responsible for chemical burning followed by sensitization in a chemistry student.

Suggested Reading
Goossens A, Deschutter A (2003) Acute irritation followed by primary sensitization to 2-cyclohenen-1-one in a chemistry student. Contact Dermatitis 48 : 163–164

120. N-Cyclohexyl-2-Benzothiazylsulfenamide

CAS Registry Number
{95–33–0]

A rubber accelerator chemical. The most frequent occupational categories are metal industry, homemakers, health services and laboratories, and the building industry.

Suggested Reading

Condé-Salazar L, Del-Rio E, Guimaraens D, Gonzalez Domingo A (1993) Type IV allergy to rubber additives: a 10-year study of 686 cases. J Am Acad Dermatol 29:176–180

Kiec-Swierczynska M (1995) Occupational sensitivity to rubber. Contact Dermatitis 32:171–172

Von Hintzenstern J, Heese A, Koch HU, Peters KP, Hornstein OP (1991) Frequency, spectrum and occupational relevance of type IV allergies to rubber chemicals. Contact Dermatitis 24:244–252

121. N-Cyclohexyl-N′-Phenyl-p-Phenylenediamine

N-Phenyl-N′-Cyclohexyl-p-Phenylenediamine, CPPD

CAS Registry Number [101–87–1]

CPPD is a rubber chemical used as an antioxidant. Cross-reactions are frequently observed with N-isopropyl-N′-phenylparaphenylenediamine (IPPD).

Suggested Reading

Hervé-Bazin B, Gradiski D, Duprat P, Marignac B, Foussereau J, Cavelier C, Bieber P (1977) Occupational eczema from N-isopropyl-N′-phenyl-paraphenylenediamine (IPPD) and N-dimethyl-1,3 butyl-N′-phenyl-paraphenylenediamine (DMPPD) in tyres. Contact Dermatitis 3:1–15

Von Hintzenstern J, Heese A, Koch HU, Peters KP, Hornstein OP (1991) Frequency, spectrum and occupational relevance of type IV allergies to rubber chemicals. Contact Dermatitis 24:244–252

84 Christophe J. Le Coz, Jean-Pierre Lepoittevin

122. *N*-Cyclohexyl-Thiophthalimide

CAS Registry Number [17796–82–6]

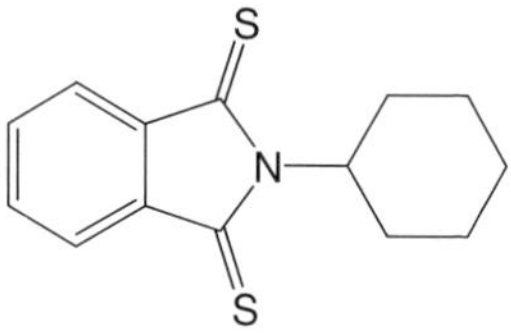

N-Cyclohexyl-thiophthalimide is a rubber chemical, widely used as a vulcanization retarder. Sensitization sources are often protective gloves.

Suggested Reading

Huygens S, Barbaud A, Goossens A (2001) Frequency and relevance of positive patch tests to cyclohexylthiophthalimide, a new rubber allergen. Eur J Dermatol 11:443–445

Kanerva L, Estlander T, Jolanki R (1996) Allergic patch test reactions caused by the rubber chemical cyclohexyl thiophthalimide. Contact Dermatitis 34:23–26

123. Cymene

Cymol, Methyl-Isopropyl-Benzol

CAS Registry Number [25155–15–1]

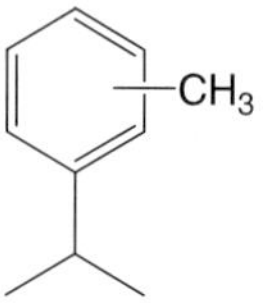

Terpenes, constitutive of essential oils, are hydrocarbons with the general formula $C_{10}H_{16}$. They are structurally related to cymol.

Suggested Reading

Selvaag E, Holm JO, Thune P (1995) Allergic contact dermatitis in an aroma therapist with multiple sensitizations to essential oils. Contact Dermatitis 33:354–355

124. Cymoxanil

2-Cyano-N-[(Ethylamino)Carbonyl]-2-(Methoxyimino)Acetamide

CAS Registry Number
[57966–95–7]

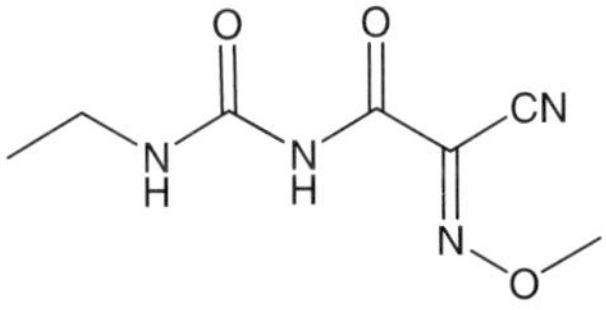

Cymoxanil, an urea derivative, is included (10%) with dithianone (25%) in Aktuan®. It is a fungicide agent, possibly sensitizing agricultural workers.

Suggested Reading
Koch P (1996) Occupational allergic contact dermatitis and airborne contact dermatitis from 5 fungicides in a vineyard worker. Cross-reactions between fungicides of the dithiocarbamate group? Contact Dermatitis 34:324–329

125. Dazomet

3,5-Dimethyltetrahydro-1,3,5(2H)Thiadiazine-2-Thione, DMTT

CAS Registry Number [533–74–4]

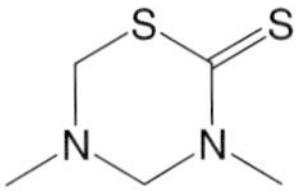

Dazomet is a biocide used to control bacterial and fungal growth in a pulp and paper system, and also in agriculture for soil disinfection. It is contained in Busan 1058, Mylone and Fungicide 974 (Crag™). Sensitization, rarely reported, occurred in a paper mill worker.

Suggested Reading
Warin AP (1992) Allergic contact dermatitis from dazomet. Contact Dermatitis 26:135–136

126. DDT

Dichlorodiphenyltrichloroethane

CAS Registry Number [50–29–3]

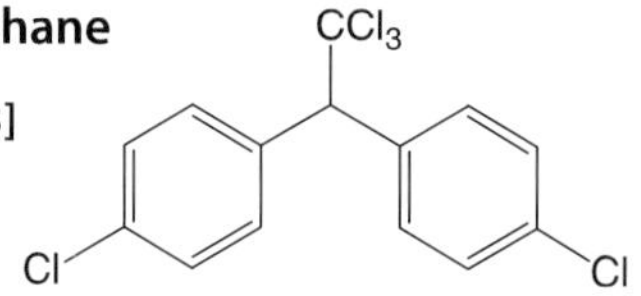

This insecticide was formerly reported as a sensitizer in farmers or agricultural workers.

Suggested Reading

Sharma VK, Kaur S (1990) Contact sensitization by pesticides in farmers. Contact Dermatitis 23:77–80

127. Decyl glucoside

CAS Registry Numbers [58846–77–8], [68515–73–1], [141464–42–8], and [54549–25–6]

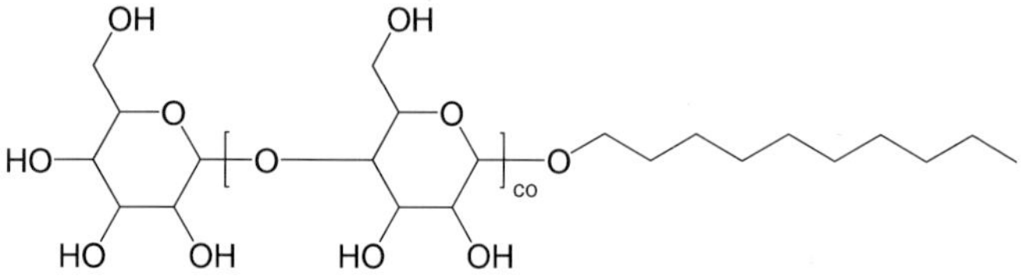

CAS : 54549-25-6   co : 1 to 3

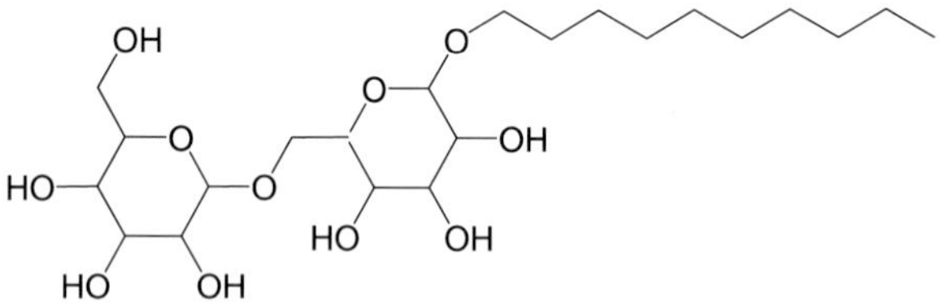

Decyl glucoside or decyl D-glucoside, also named decyl-beta-D-glucopyranoside, belongs to the alkyl glucosides family, and is obtained by condensation of the fatty alcohol decyl alcohol and a

D-glucose polymer. This nonionic surfactant and cleansing agent has been widely used for several years, due to its foaming power and good tolerance in rinse-off products such as shampoos, hair dyes and colors, and soaps. Decyl glucoside is also employed in leave-on products such as no-rinsing cleansing milks, lotions and several sunscreen agents, and is contained as a stabilizing surfactant of organic microparticles in sunscreen agent Tinosorb® M.

Suggested Reading
Blondeel A (2003) Contact allergy to the mild surfactant decylglucoside. Contact Dermatitis 49:304–305
Le Coz CJ, Meyer MT (2003) Contact allergy to decyl glucoside in antiseptic after body piercing. Contact Dermatitis 48:279–280

128. Dehydrocostuslactone

CAS Registry Number [477–43–0]

A guaianolide sesquiterpene lactone extracted from costus oil. It is one of the components of Lactone mix, with costunolide and alantolactone, used to detect Compositae-sensitive patients.

Suggested Reading
Ducombs G, Benezra C, Talaga P, Andersen KE, Burrows D, Camarasa JG, Dooms-Goossens A, Frosch PJ, Lachapelle JM, Menné T, Rycroft RJG, White IR, Shaw S, Wilkinson JD (1990) Patch testing with the "sesquiterpene lactone mix": a marker for contact allergy to Compositae and other sesquiterpene-lactone-containing plants. Contact Dermatitis 22:249–252

129. Deoxylapachol

CAS Registry Number [3568–90–9]

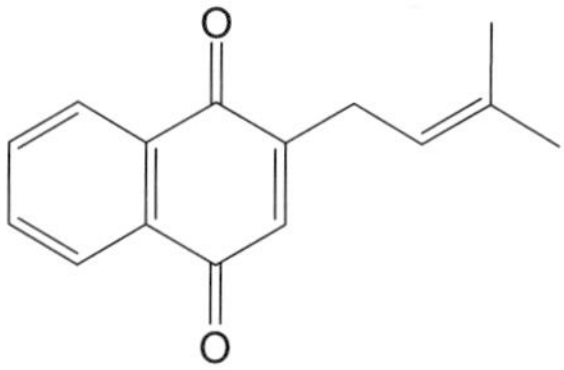

Deoxylapachol is the main allergen identified in teak (*Tectona grandis*). Sensitization often concerns people involved in woodwork.

Suggested Reading

Lamminpää A, Estlander T, Jolanki R, Kanerva L (1996) Occupational allergic contact dermatitis caused by decorative plants. Contact Dermatitis 34:330–335
Meding B, Ahman M, Karlberg AT (1996) Skin symptoms and contact allergy in woodwork teachers. Contact Dermatitis 34:185–190

130. Diallyl Disulfide

CAS Registry Number [2179–57–9]

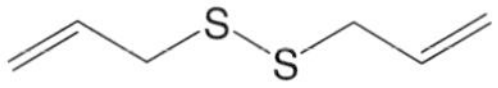

Diallyl disulfide is one of the major allergens in garlic (*Allium sativum*) and onions. Among patients patch-test-positive to garlic, all 13 who were tested had positive reactions to diallyl sulfide 5% pet.

Suggested Reading

Bruynzeel DP (1997) Bulb dermatitis. Dermatological problems in the flower bulb industries. Contact Dermatitis 37:70–77
Lamminpää A, Estlander T, Jolanki R, Kanerva L (1996) Occupational allergic contact dermatitis caused by decorative plants. Contact Dermatitis 34:330–335
McFadden JP, White IR, Rycroft RJG (1992) Allergic contact dermatitis from garlic. Contact Dermatitis 27:333–334

131. Diaminodiphenylmethane

4,4'-Diaminodiphenylmethane, 4,4'-Methylenedianiline

CAS Registry Number [107–77–9]

4,4'-Diaminodiphenylmethane is an aromatic diamine used as a curing agent in epoxy resins of the bisphenol A type, and in the production of plastics, isocyanates, adhesives, elastomers, polyurethane (elastic and rigid foams, paints, lacquers, adhesives, binding agents, synthetics rubbers, and elastomeric fibres), and butyl rubber. 4,4'-Diaminodiphenylmethane is also a by-product in azo dyes. It is also possibly formed by hydrolysis of diphenylmethane-4,4'-diisocyanate.

Suggested Reading

Bruynzeel DP, van der Wegen-Keijser MH (1993) Contact dermatitis in a cast technician. Contact Dermatitis 28:193–194

Condé-Salazar L, Gonzalez de Domingo MA, Guimaraens D (1994) Sensitization to epoxy resin systems in special flooring workers. Contact Dermatitis 31:157–160

Holness DL, Nethercott JR (1993) The performance of specialized collections of bisphenol A epoxy resin system components in the evaluation of workers in an occupational health clinic population. Contact Dermatitis 28:216–219

Jolanki R, Kanerva L, Estlander T, Tarvainen K, Keskinen H, Henriks-Eckerman ML (1990) Occupational dermatoses from epoxy resin compounds. Contact Dermatitis 23:172–183

Jolanki R, Kanerva L, Estlander T, Tarvainen K (1994) Concomitant sensitization to triglycidyl isocyanurate, diaminodiphenylmethane and 2-hydroxyethyl methacrylate from silk-screen printing coatings in the manufacture of circuit boards. Contact Dermatitis 30:12–15

Kiec-Swierczynska M (1995) Rubber chemical. Occupational sensitivity to rubber. Contact Dermatitis 32:171–172

Mancuso G, Reggiani M, Berdondini RM (1996) Occupational dermatitis in shoemakers. Contact Dermatitis 34:17–22

Tarvainen K (1995) Analysis of patients with allergic patch test reactions to a plastic and glues series. Contact Dermatitis 32:346–351

132. Diammonium Hydrogen Phosphate

CAS Registry Number [7783–28–0]

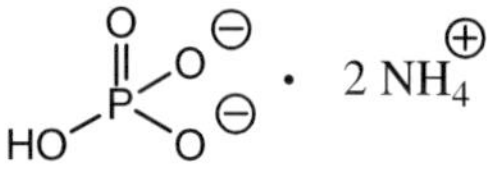

$$\text{HO}-\overset{\displaystyle O}{\underset{\displaystyle O^{\ominus}}{\overset{\|}{P}}}-O^{\ominus} \quad \cdot \quad 2\,\text{NH}_4^{\oplus}$$

A flame retardant which caused contact dermatitis in surgical personnel. It was due to excessive residual concentrations in surgical garbs.

Suggested Reading

Belsito DV (1990) Contact dermatitis from diammonium hydrogen phosphate in surgical garb. Contact Dermatitis 23:267–268

133. Diazodiethylaniline Chloride

CAS Registry Number
[148–90–3]

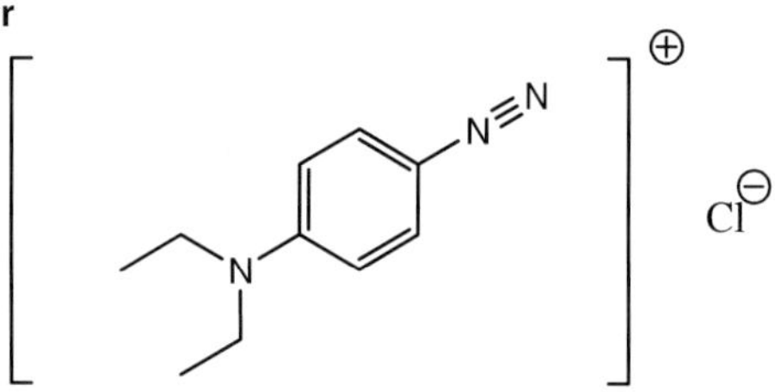

It is a well-known allergen in diazo copy paper. This product is allergenic until exposed to light, and inactivated by UV radiations.

Suggested Reading

Foussereau J, Benezra C (1970) Les eczémas allergiques professionnels. Masson, Paris

Pambor M, Poweleit H (1992) Allergic contact dermatitis due to diazo copy paper. Contact Dermatitis 26:131–132

134. Diazolidinyl Urea

Germall II

CAS Registry Number
[78491–02–8]

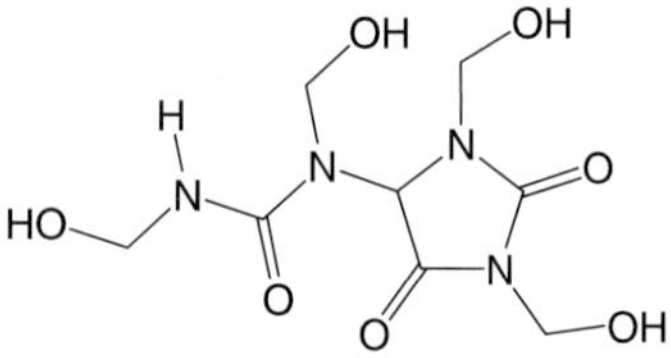

Diazolidinyl urea, a formaldehyde releaser, is contained mainly in cosmetics and toiletries, and can be found in barrier creams.

Suggested Reading

Le Coz CJ (2005) Hypersensibilité à la Diazolidinyl urée et à l'Imidazolidinyl urée. Ann Dermatol Venereol 132 (in press)

Van Hecke E, Suys E (1994) Where next to look for formaldehyde? Contact Dermatitis 31:268

135. Dibenzothiazyl Disulfide

CAS Registry Number
[120–78–5]

This rubber chemical of the mercaptobenzothiazole group is used as a vulcanization accelerant. The most frequent occupational categories are metal industry, homemakers, health services and laboratories, and the building industry.

Suggested Reading

Condé-Salazar L, Del-Rio E, Guimaraens D, Gonzalez Domingo A (1993) Type IV allergy to rubber additives: a 10-year study of 686 cases. J Am Acad Dermatol 29:176–180

Le Coz CJ (2004) Fiche d'éviction en cas d'hypersensibilité au mercaptobenzothiazole et au mercapto mix. Ann Dermatol Venereol 131:846–848

Von Hintzenstern J, Heese A, Koch HU, Peters KP, Hornstein OP (1991) Frequency, spectrum and occupational relevance of type IV allergies to rubber chemicals. Contact Dermatitis 24:244–252

136. Dibucaine (Hydrochloride)

Cincaine, Cinchocain(e), Percaine, Sovcaine

CAS Registry Number [85–79–0] (CAS Registry Number [61–12–1])

• HCl

Dibucaine hydrochloride is an amide group local anesthetic that can induce allergic contact dermatitis.

Suggested Reading
Erdmann SM, Sachs B, Merk HF (2001) Systemic contact dermatitis from cinchocaine. Contact Dermatitis 44:260–261
Nakada T, Iijima M (2000) Allergic contact dermatitis from dibucaine hydrochloride. Contact Dermatitis 42:283

137. Dibutyl Phthalate

CAS Registry Number [84–74–2]

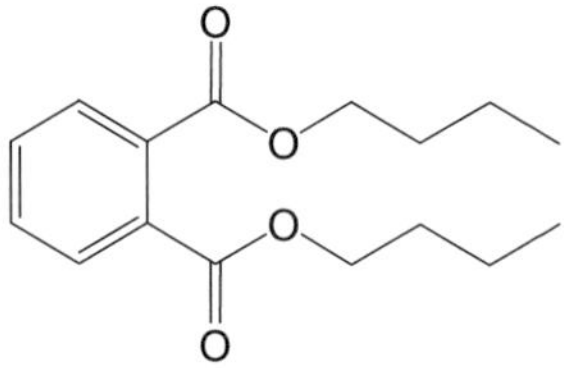

It is mainly used as a nonreactive epoxy diluent.

Suggested Reading
Capon F, Cambie MP, Clinard F, Bernardeau K, Kalis B (1996) Occupational contact dermatitis caused by computer mice. Contact Dermatitis 35:57–58
Chieregato C, Vincenzi C, Guerra L, Farina P (1994) Occupational allergic contact dermatitis due to ethylenediamine dihydrochloride and cresyl glycidyl ether in epoxy resin systems. Contact Dermatitis 30:120

138. Dibutylthiourea

1,3-Dibutyl-2-Thiourea

CAS Registry Number [109–46–6]

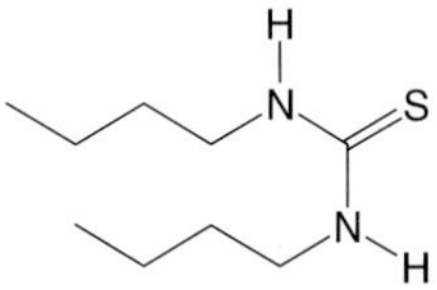

Dibutylthiourea is used in the vulcanization of rubber, in paints and glue removers as an anticorrosive, in phonecards as a component of the thermocoating sprayed over the optically read layer of the card. Cross sensitivity to other thiourea derivatives is possible.

Suggested Reading

Kanerva L, Estlander T, Jolanki R (1994) Occupational allergic contact dermatitis caused by thiourea compounds. Contact Dermatitis 31: 242–248

Kiec-Swierczynska M (1995) Occupational sensitivity to rubber. Contact Dermatitis 32:171–172

Schmid-Grendelmeier P, Elsner P (1995) Contact dermatitis due to occupational dibutylthiourea exposure: a case of phonecard dermatitis. Contact Dermatitis 32:308–309

139. 4,5-Dichloro-2-*n*-Octyl-4-Isothiazolin-3-one

Kathon® 930

CAS Registry Number [64359–81–5]

Irritant and sensitizer, Kathon® 930 caused contact dermatitis in employees of a textile finishing factory.

Suggested Reading

Kawai K, Nagakawa M, Sasaki Y, Kawai Y (1993) Occupational contact dermatitis from Kathon® 930. Contact Dermatitis 28:117–118

140. 1,3-Dichloropropene

1,3-Dichloro-1-Prop(yl)ene, 1,3-Dichloro-2-Prop(yl)ene, DD-95

CAS Registry Number [542–75–6]

This nematocide is used as a soil fumigant prior to crop cultivation. Farmers and process operators employed at pesticide plants are mainly exposed.

Suggested Reading

Bousema MT, Wiemer GR, van Joost T (1991) A classic case of sensitization to DD-95. Contact Dermatitis 24:132

141. Dichlorvos

CAS Registry Number [62–73–7]

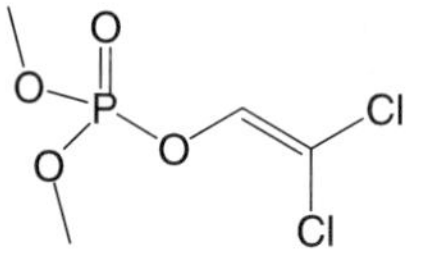

Cases of sensitization to this organophosphorus compound with several commercial names (Benfos, Brevinyl, Chlorvinphos, DDVP, Equigard, Fly fighte, Nogos, and Unifos), were occupationally seen in chrysanthem growers, horticulturists, technicians, and in a chemist.

Suggested Reading

Cleenewerck MB, Martin P (1990) Dermite de contact au Dichlorvos. Rev Fr Allergol 30 : 38

Mathias CG (1983) Persistent contact dermatitis from the insecticide dichlorvos. Contact Dermatitis 9 : 217–218

142. *N,N*-Dicyclohexyl-2-Benzothiazole Sulfenamide

CAS Registry Number [4979–32–2]

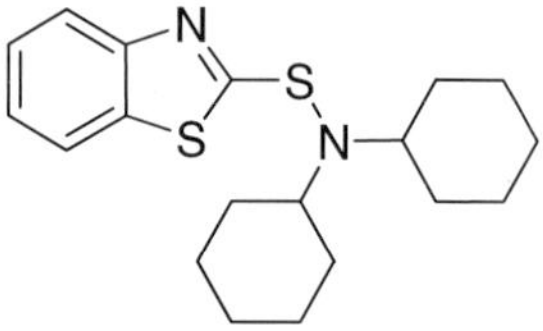

This substance is a rubber accelerator of the mercaptobenzothiazole-sulfenamide group.

Suggested Reading

Le Coz CJ (2004) Fiche d'éviction en cas d'hypersensibilité au mercapto-benzothiazole et au mercapto mix. Ann Dermatol Venereol 131 : 846–848

143. Dicyclohexyl Carbodiimide

CAS Registry Number
[538–75–0]

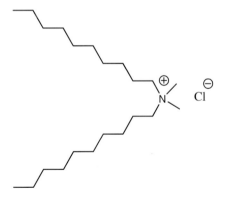

Used in peptide chemistry as a coupling reagent. It is both an irritant and a sensitizer, and has caused contact dermatitis in pharmacists and chemists.

Suggested Reading
Poesen N, de Moor A, Busschots A, Dooms-Goossens A (1995) Contact allergy to dicyclohexyl carbodiimide and diisopropyl carbodiimide. Contact Dermatitis 32:368–369

144. Didecyldimethylammonium Chloride

Bardac-22

CAS Registry Number
[7173–51–5]

This quaternary ammonium compound is used as a detergent-disinfectant in hospitals, as an algaecide in swimming pools, as a fungicide, and against termites in wood. We recently observed severe contact dermatitis in a slaughterhouse worker using a liquid soap containing this product (personal observation).

Suggested Reading
Dejobert Y, Martin P, Piette F, Thomas P, Bergoend H (1997) Contact
    dermatitis from didecyldimethylammonium chloride and bis-(amino-
    propyl)-laurylamine in a detergent-disinfectant used in hospital.
    Contact Dermatitis 37 : 95–96

145. Diethanolamine

CAS Registry Number [111–42–2]

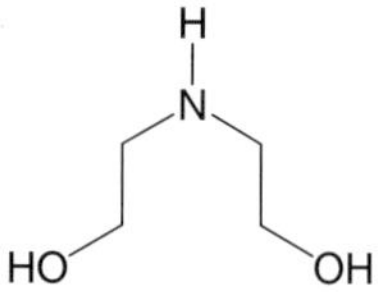

Diethanolamine is contained in many products, as a metalworking
fluid. Traces may exist in other ethanolamine-containing fluids.

Suggested Reading
Blum A, Lischka G (1997) Allergic contact dermatitis from mono-, di- and
    triethanolamine. Contact Dermatitis 36 : 166

146. Diethyl Sebacate

Ethyl Sebacate, Diethyl Decanedioate

CAS Registry Number [110–40–7]

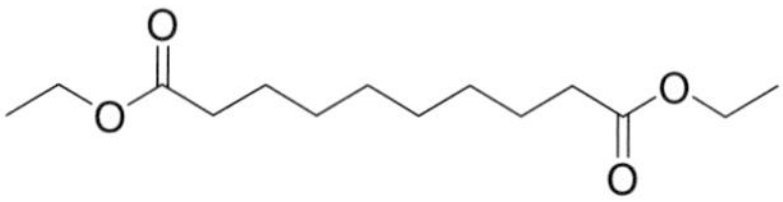

This emulsifier has rarely been reported as a sensitizing agent,
mainly in topical treatments.

Suggested Reading
Tanaka M, Kobayashi S, Murata T, Tanikawa A, Nishikawa T (2000) Aller-
    gic contact dermatitis from diethyl sebacate in lanoconazole cream.
    Contact Dermatitis 43 : 233–234

147. Diethyleneglycol Diglycidyl Ether

Ether, bis[2-(2,3-Epoxypropoxy)Ethyl]

CAS Registry Number [4206–61–5]

Diethyleneglycol diglycidyl ether was contained in a reactive diethyleneglycol-based diluent of epoxy resins and caused contact dermatitis in three workers at a ski factory.

Suggested Reading

Jolanki R, Tarvainen K, Tatar T, Estlander T, Henriks-Eckerman ML, Mustakallio KK, Kanerva L (1996) Occupational dermatoses from exposure to epoxy resin compounds in a ski factory. Contact Dermatitis 34:390–396

148. Diethylenetriamine

CAS Registry Number [111–40–0]

Diethylenetriamine is a hardener in epoxy resins of the Bisphenol A type. It has been reported to be a sensitizer when used in an ultrasonic bath for cleaning jewels, in synthetic lubricants or in carbonless copy paper.

Suggested Reading

Holness DL, Nethercott JR (1993) The performance of specialized collections of bisphenol A epoxy resin system components in the evaluation of workers in an occupational health clinic population. Contact Dermatitis 28:216–219

Jolanki R, Kanerva L, Estlander T, Tarvainen K, Keskinen H, Henriks-Eckerman ML (1990) Occupational dermatoses from epoxy resin compounds. Contact Dermatitis 23:172–183

Kanerva L, Estlander T, Jolanki R (1990) Occupational allergic contact dermatitis due to diethylenetriamine (DETA) from carbonless copy paper and from an epoxy compound. Contact Dermatitis 23:272–273

149. Diethylphthalate

CAS Registry Number [84–66–2]

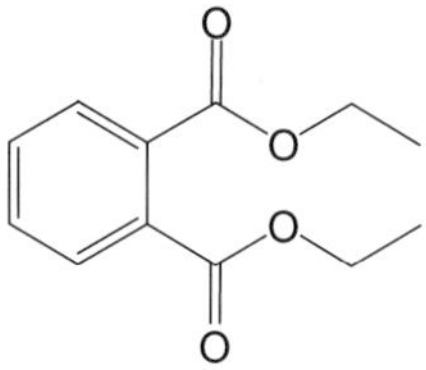

This plasticizer increases the flexibility of plastics. It is also contained in deodorant formulations, perfumes, emollients, and insect repellents. It can cross react with dimethyl phthalate.

Suggested Reading
Capon F, Cambie MP, Clinard F, Bernardeau K, Kalis B (1996) Occupational contact dermatitis caused by computer mice. Contact Dermatitis 35:57–58

150. Diethylthiourea

Diethylthiocarbamide

CAS Registry Number [105–55–5]

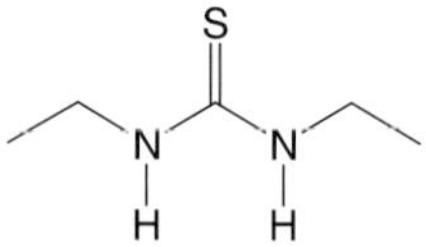

Diethylthiourea, a thiourea derivative, is used mainly as a rubber chemical, particularly in solid neoprene products.

Suggested Reading
Kanerva L, Estlander T, Jolanki R (1994) Occupational allergic contact dermatitis caused by thiourea compounds. Contact Dermatitis 31: 242–248

151. Diisopropyl Carbodiimide

N,N′-Methanetetraylbis-2-Propanamine

CAS Registry Number [693–13–0]

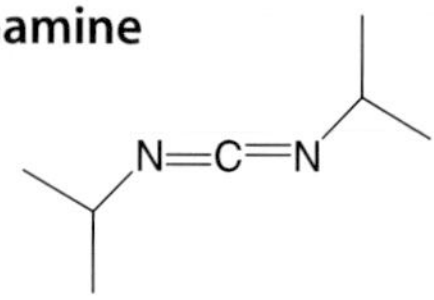

It is used in peptide chemistry as a coupling reagent. It is very toxic and causes contact dermatitis in laboratory workers.

Suggested Reading

Poesen N, de Moor A, Busschots A, Dooms-Goossens A (1995) Contact allergy to dicyclohexyl carbodiimide and diisopropyl carbodiimide. Contact Dermatitis 32:368–369

152. Diisopropylbenzothiazyl-2-Sulfenamide

CAS Registry Number [95–29–4]

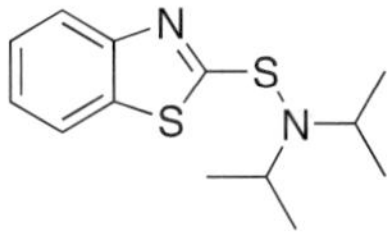

This chemical is a mercaptobenzothiazole-sulfenamide used in rubber vulcanization.

Suggested Reading

Le Coz CJ (2004) Fiche d'éviction en cas d'hypersensibilité au mercaptobenzothiazole et au mercapto mix. Ann Dermatol Venereol 131: 846–848

153. 2,5-Dimercapto-1,3,4-Thiadiazole

DMTD

CAS Registry Number [1072–71–5]

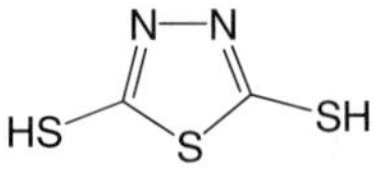

This low-molecular-weight aromatic compound is used in the production of copper corrosion inhibitors for engine oils, flame retardants, and photographic development chemicals. Seven cases of industrial allergic sensitization were reported in a manufacturing plant.

Suggested Reading

O'Driscoll JO, Beck M, Taylor S (1990) Occupational contact allergy to 2,5-dimercapto-1,3,4-thiadiazole. Contact Dermatitis 23:268–269

154. Dimethoate

CAS Registry Number [60–51–5]

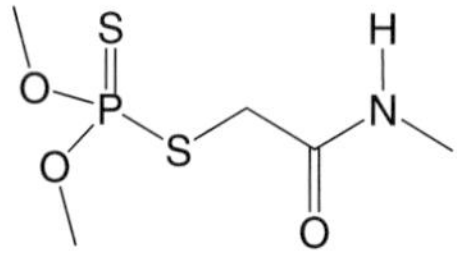

This organophosphorus compound is used as a contact and systemic insecticide and acaricide. It induced an erythema-multi-form-like contact dermatitis in a warehouseman in an agricultural consortium.

Suggested Reading
Haenen C, de Moor A, Dooms-Goossens A (1996) Contact dermatitis caused by the insecticides omethoate and dimethoate. Contact Dermatitis 35:54–55
Schena D, Barba A (1992) Erythema-multiforme-like contact dermatitis from dimethoate. Contact Dermatitis 27:116–117

155. Dimethoxon

Omethoate

CAS Registry Number [1113–02–6]

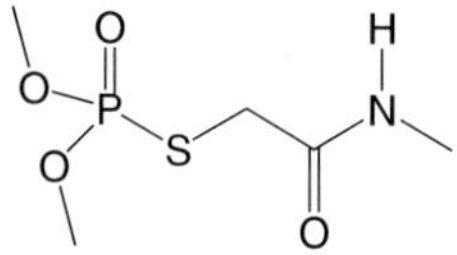

Contact dermatitis from omethoate–dimethoxon is rare.

Suggested Reading
De Moor A, Dooms-Goossens A (1996) Contact dermatitis caused by the insecticides omethoate and dimethoate. Contact Dermatitis 35:54–55

156. 2,6-Dimethoxy-1,4-Benzoquinone

CAS Registry Number [530–55–2]

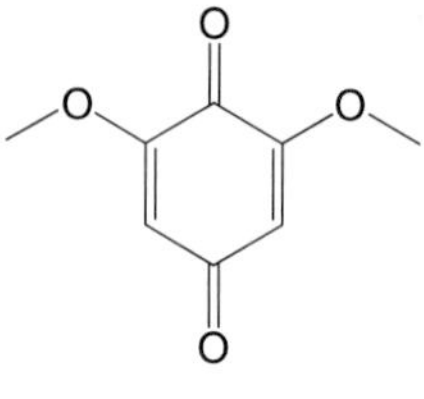

2,6-Dimethoxy-1,4-benzoquinone is an allergen in more than 50 different plants and wood species, e.g., mahogany, macore, sipo, wenge, oak, beech, elms, and poplar. With acamelin, it is one of the allergens of *Acacia melanoxylon*. Sensitization can occur in woodworkers such as carpenters, joiners, and sawyers.

Suggested Reading

Correia O, Barros MA, Mesquita-Guimaraes J (1992) Airborne contact dermatitis from the woods *Acacia melanoxylon* and *Entandophragma cylindricum*. Contact Dermatitis 27:343–344

Lamminpää A, Estlander T, Jolanki R, Kanerva L (1996) Occupational allergic contact dermatitis caused by decorative plants. Contact Dermatitis 34:330–335

157. (*R*)-3,4-Dimethoxy-Dalbergione

CAS Registry Number [37555–64–4]

This quinone is the main allergen of *Machaerium scleroxylum* Tul. (Santos rosewood, *Pao ferro*, *Caviuna vermelha*, *Santos palissander*). Occupational sensitization mainly concerns woodworkers.

Suggested Reading

Chieregato C, Vincenzi C, Guerra L, Rapacchiale S (1993) Occupational airborne contact dermatitis from *Machaerium scleroxylum* (Santos rosewood). Contact Dermatitis 29:164–165

Lamminpää A, Estlander T, Jolanki R, Kanerva L (1996) Occupational allergic contact dermatitis caused by decorative plants. Contact Dermatitis 34:330–335

158. (S)-4,4'-Dimethoxy Dalbergione

CAS Registry Number [4646–87–1]

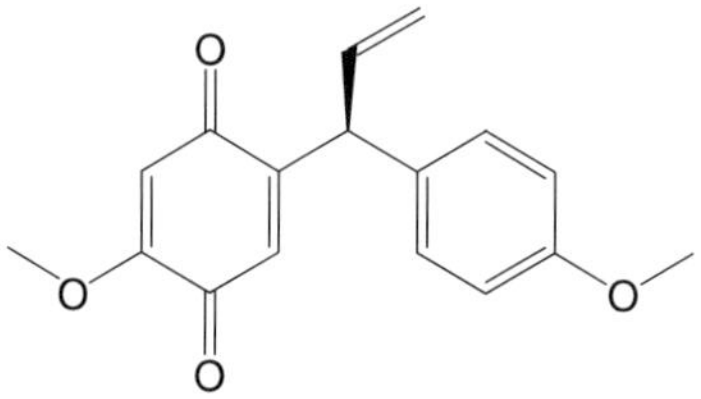

It is an allergen of *Dalbergia nigra* also contained in *Dalbergia latifolia* Roxb. (East Indian rosewood, palissander). Occupational dermatitis can occur in timberworkers such as carpenters, sawyers, joiners or knifegrinders.

Suggested Reading

Gallo R, Guarrera M, Hausen BM (1996) Airborne contact dermatitis from East Indian rosewood (*Dalbergia latifolia* Roxb.). Contact Dermatitis 35:60–61

159. 5,8-Dimethoxypsoralen

Isopimpinellin

CAS Registry Number [482–27–9]

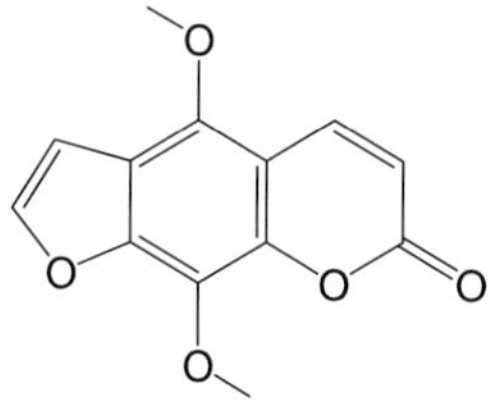

Psoralens are natural photoactivable compounds in plants and can cause phototoxic contact dermatitis. For example, *Cachrys libanotis* L., Apiaceae-Umbelliferae family, contains 5,8-dimethoxypsoralen.

Suggested Reading

Ena P, Cerri R, Dessi G, Manconi PM, Atzei AD (1991) Phototoxicity due to *Cachrys libanotis*. Contact Dermatitis 24:1–5

160. Dimethyl Phthalate

CAS Registry Number [131–11–3]

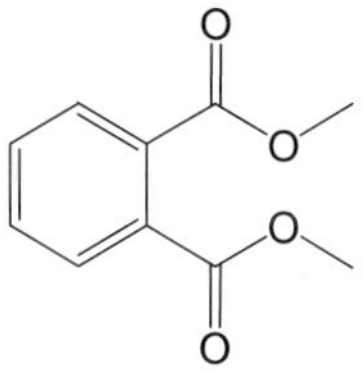

Phthalates are plasticizers, and increase the flexibility of plastics. They are also found in deodorant formulations, perfumes, emollients, and insect repellents.

Suggested Reading

Capon F, Cambie MP, Clinard F, Bernardeau K, Kalis B (1996) Occupational contact dermatitis caused by computer mice. Contact Dermatitis 35:57–58

161. 4-N,N-(Dimethylamino) Benzenediazonium Chloride

p-Diazodimethylaniline zinc Chloride Double Salt

CAS Registry Number [100–04–9]

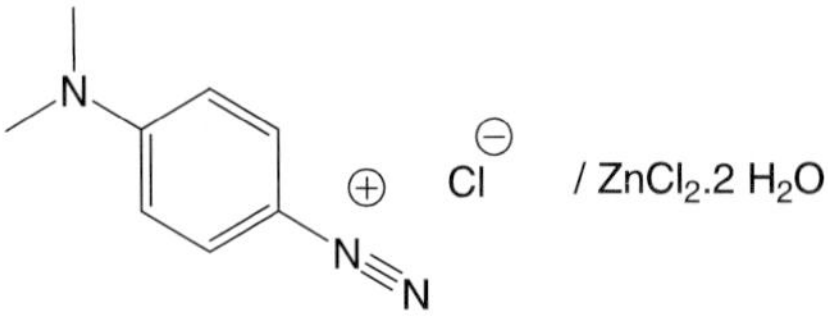

It is a diazo compound found in diazo copy paper. It is allergenic only when unexposed.

Suggested Reading

Geier J, Fuchs T (1993) Contact allergy due to 4-N,N-dimethylaminobenzene diazonium chloride and thiourea in diazo copy paper. Contact Dermatitis 28:304–305

162. 3-Dimethylaminopropylamine

CAS Registry Number [109–55–7]

Dimethylaminopropylamine is an aliphatic amine present in ampho-teric surfactants such as liquid soaps and shampoos. It is present as a residual impurity thought to be responsible for allergy from cocamidopropylbetaine. It is structurally similar to diethyl-aminopropylamine. It is also used as a curing agent for epoxy resins and an organic intermediate in chemical synthesises (ion exchangers, additives for flocculants, cosmetics and fuel additives, dyes and pesticides). Patch test has to be carefully interpreted, since the 1% aqueous solution has pH>11 (personal observation).

Suggested Reading

Angelini G, Foti C, Rigano L, Vena GA (1995) 3-Dimethylaminopropyl-amine: a key substance in contact allergy to cocamidopropylbetaine? Contact Dermatitis 32:96–99
Kanerva L, Estlander T, Jolanki R (1996) Occupational allergic contact dermatitis from 3-dimethylaminopropylamine in shampoos. Contact Dermatitis 35:122–123
Speight EL, Beck MH, Lawrence CM (1993) Occupational allergic contact dermatitis due to 3-dimethylaminopropylamine. Contact Dermatitis 28:49–50

163. Dimethyldiphenylthiuram disulfide

CAS Registry Number [53880–86–7]

This thiuram compound is used as an accelerator for rubber vulcanization.

Suggested Reading

Le Coz CJ (2004) Fiche d'éviction en cas d'hypersensibilité au thiuram mix. Ann Dermatol Venereol 131:1012–1014

164. Dimethylformamide

CAS Registry Number [68–12–2]

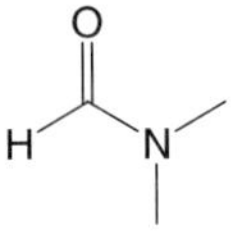

This is an organic solvent for vinyl resins and acetylene, butadiene and acid gases. It caused contact dermatitis in a technician at an epoxy resin factory, and can provoke alcohol-induced flushing in exposed subjects.

Suggested Reading

Camarasa JG (1987) Contact dermatitis from dimethylformamide. Contact Dermatitis 16:234

Cox NH, Mustchin CP (1991) Prolonged spontaneous and alcohol-induced flushing due to the solvent dimethyl formamide. Contact Dermatitis 24 :69–70

165. 2,4-Dimethylol Phenol

CAS Registry Number [2937–60–2]

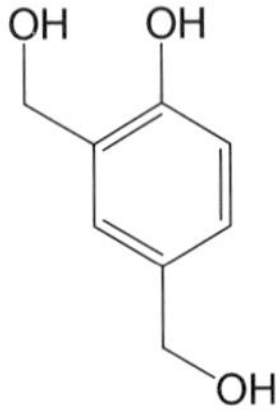

2,4-Dimethylol phenol in a compound of resins based on phenol and formaldehyde. Cross-reactivity is possible with other phenol derivative molecules.

Suggested Reading

Bruze M, Zimerson E (1997) Cross-reaction patterns in patients with contact allergy to simple methylol phenols. Contact Dermatitis 37:82–86

Bruze M, Zimerson E (1985) Contact allergy to 3-methylol phenol, 2,4-dimethylol phenol and 2,6-dimethylol phenol. Acta Derm Venereol (Stockh) 65:548–551

166. 2,6-Dimethylol Phenol

CAS Registry Number [2937–59–9]

This substance is contained in resins based on phenol and formaldehyde. Cross-reactivity is possible with other phenol derivative molecules.

Suggested Reading

Bruze M, Zimerson E (1985) Contact allergy to 3-methylol phenol, 2,4-dimethylol phenol and 2,6-dimethylol phenol. Acta Derm Venereol (Stockh) 65:548–551
Bruze M, Zimerson E (1997) Cross-reaction patterns in patients with contact allergy to simple methylol phenols. Contact Dermatitis 37:82–86

167. Dimethylthiourea

Dimethylthiocarbamide

CAS Registry Number [534–13–4]

Dimethylthiocarbamide, an antioxygen agent, is responsible for sensitization, when unexposed to light, from diazo papers.

Suggested Reading

Geier J, Fuchs T (1993) Contact allergy due to 4-N,N-dimethylamino-benzene diazonium chloride and thiourea in diazo copy paper. Contact Dermatitis 28:304–305
Kanerva L, Estlander T, Jolanki R (1994) Occupational allergic contact dermatitis caused by thiourea compounds. Contact Dermatitis 31:242–248

168. Dinitrochlorobenzene

DNCB, 2,4-Dinitrochlorobenzene,
2,4-Dinitro-1-Chlorobenzene,
4-Chloro-1,3-Dinitrobenzene, 6-Chloro-1,3-Dinitrobenzene

CAS Registry Number [97–00–7]

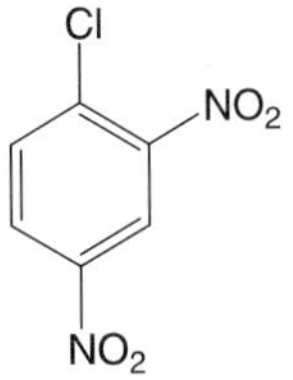

This substance is one of the strongest primary skin irritant known, and a universal contact allergen. Occupational dermatitis has been reported, but current use is decreasing or performed with completely closed systems. DNCB is sometimes used for topical treatment of alopecia areata, severe warts, and cutaneous metastasis of malignant melanoma.

Suggested Reading
Adams RM, Zimmerman MC, Bartlett JB, Preston JF (1971) 1-Chloro-2,4-dinitrobenzene as an algicide. Report of four cases of contact dermatitis. Arch Dermatol 103:191–193

169. Dinitrofluorobenzene

DNFB, FDNB, 2,4-Dinitro-1-Fluorobenzene, Sanger's Reagent

CAS Registry Number [70–34–8]

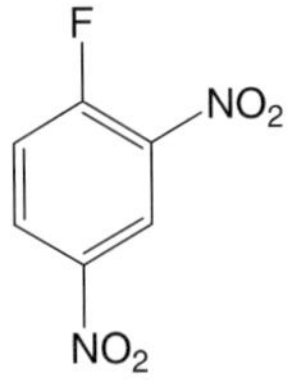

DNFB is a strong skin irritant and a universal contact allergen. It is used as an intermediate in the synthesis of pesticides and pharmaceuticals such as flurbiprofen, a chemical reagent, and as a topical sensitizer for treatment of alopecia areata.

Suggested Reading
Perez A, Narayan S, Sansom J (2004) Occupational contact dermatitis from 2,4-dinitrofluorobenzene. Contact Dermatitis 51:314

170. 2,4-Dinitrotoluene

CAS Registry Number [121–14–12]

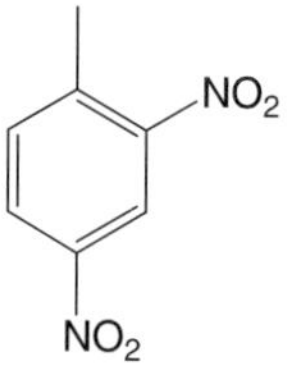

Dinitrotoluene induced sensitization in a worker for an explosives manufacturer, also sensitized to nitroglycerin.

Suggested Reading

Kanerva L, Laine R, Jolanki R, Tarvainen K, Estlander T, Helander I (1991) Occupational allergic contact dermatitis caused by nitroglycerin. Contact Dermatitis 24:356–362

171. Dipentamethylenethiuram Disulfide

CAS Registry Number [94–37–1}

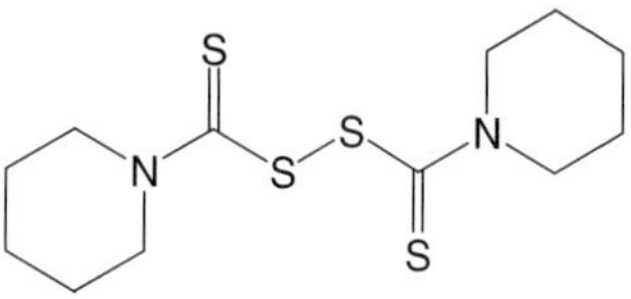

A rubber chemical contained in "thiuram mix." The most frequent occupational categories are the metal industry, homemakers, health services and laboratories, and the building industry.

Suggested Reading

Condé-Salazar L, Del-Rio E, Guimaraens D, Gonzalez Domingo A (1993) Type IV allergy to rubber additives: a 10-year study of 686 cases. J Am Acad Dermatol 29:176–180

Condé-Salazar L, Guimaraens D, Villegas C, Romero A, Gonzalez MA (1995) Occupational allergic contact dermatitis in construction workers. Contact Dermatitis 35:226–230

Kiec-Swierczynska M (1995) Occupational sensitivity to rubber. Contact Dermatitis 32:171–172

Von Hintzenstern J, Heese A, Koch HU, Peters KP, Hornstein OP (1991) Frequency, spectrum and occupational relevance of type IV allergies to rubber chemicals. Contact Dermatitis 24:244–252

172. Dipentamethylenethiuram Hexasulfide

CAS Registry Number [971–15–3]

This thiuram compound is used as an accelerator for rubber vulcanization.

Suggested Reading
Le Coz CJ (2004) Fiche d'éviction en cas d'hypersensibilité au thiuram mix. Ann Dermatol Venereol 131:1012–1014

173. Dipentamethylenethiuram Tetrasulfide

CAS Registry Number [120–54–7]

Dipentamethylenethiuram tetrasulfide is a thiuram compound used as an accelerator for rubber vulcanization.

Suggested Reading
Le Coz CJ (2004) Fiche d'éviction en cas d'hypersensibilité au thiuram mix. Ann Dermatol Venereol 131:1012–1014

174. Dipentene

CAS Registry Number [138–86–3]

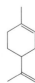

Dipentene corresponds to a racemic mixture of D-limonene and L-limonene. Dipentene can be prepared from wood turpentine or by synthesis. It is used as a solvent for waxes, rosin and gums, in printing inks, perfumes, rubber compounds, paints, enamels, and lacquers. An irritant and sensitizer, dipentene caused contact dermatitis mainly in painters, polishers, and varnishers.

Suggested Reading
Martins C, Gonçalo M, Gonçalo S (1995) Allergic contact dermatitis from dipentene in wax polish. Contact Dermatitis 33:126–127
Moura C, Dias M, Vale T (1994) Contact dermatitis in painters, polishers and varnishers. Contact Dermatitis 31:51–53

175. Diphencyprone

2,3-Diphenylcyclopropenone

CAS Registry Number [886-38-4]

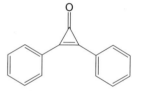

Diphencyprone is a potent contact allergen used in topical immunotherapy, to treat some severe alopecia areata. It is responsible for occupational contact dermatitis in chemists and dermatology department staff.

Suggested Reading
Sansom JE, Molloy KC, Lovell CR (1995) Occupational sensitization to diphencyprone in a chemist. Contact Dermatitis 32:363
Temesvári E, González R, Marschalkó M, Horváth A (2004) Age dependence of diphenylcyclopropenone sensitization in patients with alopecia areata. Contact Dermatitis 50:381–382

176. *N,N'*-Diphenyl-4-Phenylenediamine

DPPD

CAS Registry Number [74–31–7]

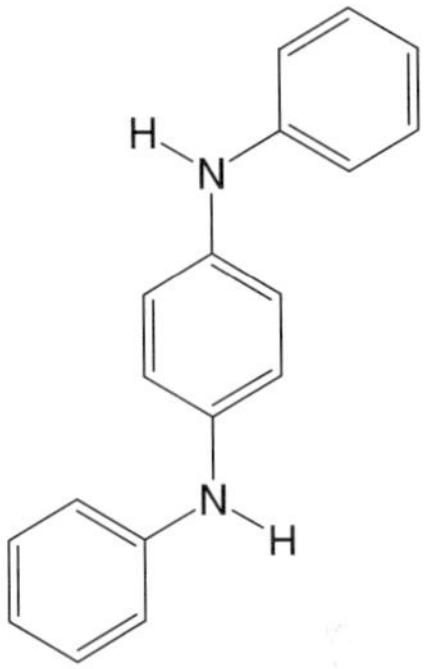

A rubber accelerant, formerly contained in "black-rubber mix." The most frequent occupational categories are in the metal industry, homemakers, health services and laboratories, and the building industry.

Suggested Reading

Condé-Salazar L, Del-Rio E, Guimaraens D, Gonzalez Domingo A (1993) Type IV allergy to rubber additives: a 10-year study of 686 cases. J Am Acad Dermatol 29:176–180

Kiec-Swierczynska M (1995) Occupational sensitivity to rubber. Contact Dermatitis 32:171–172

Von Hintzenstern J, Heese A, Koch HU, Peters KP, Hornstein OP (1991) Frequency, spectrum and occupational relevance of type IV allergies to rubber chemicals. Contact Dermatitis 24:244–252

177. 1,3-Diphenylguanidine

CAS Registry Number [102–06–7]

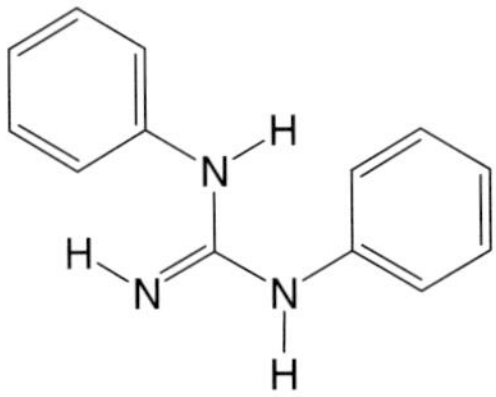

Diphenylguanidine is a rubber sensitizer that can induce immediate-type reactions and delayed-type contact allergy. It was formerly contained in "carba mix." Occupational exposure concerns finished rubber items and the rubber manufacturing industry. The most frequent occupational categories are metal industry, homemakers, health services and laboratories, and the building industry.

Suggested Reading

Bruze M, Kestrup L (1994) Occupational allergic contact dermatitis from diphenylguanidine in a gas mask. Contact Dermatitis 31:125–126

Condé-Salazar L, Del-Rio E, Guimaraens D, Gonzalez Domingo A (1993) Type IV allergy to rubber additives: a 10-year study of 686 cases. J Am Acad Dermatol 29:176–180

Kiec-Swierczynska M (1995) Occupational sensitivity to rubber. Contact Dermatitis 32:171–172

Mancuso G, Reggiani M, Berdondini RM (1996) Occupational dermatitis in shoemakers. Contact Dermatitis 34:17–22

Von Hintzenstern J, Heese A, Koch HU, Peters KP, Hornstein OP (1991) Frequency, spectrum and occupational relevance of type IV allergies to rubber chemicals. Contact Dermatitis 24:244–252

178. 4,4′-Diphenylmethane-Diisocyanate

MDI

CAS Registry Number
[101–68–8]

MDI is used in the manufacture of various polyurethane products: elastic and rigid foams, paints, lacquers, adhesives, binding agents, synthetic rubbers, and elastomeric fibers.

Suggested Reading

Estlander T, Keskinen H, Jolanki R, Kanerva L (1992) Occupational dermatitis from exposure to polyurethane chemicals. Contact Dermatitis 27:161–165

Mancuso G, Reggiani M, Berdondini RM (1996) Occupational dermatitis in shoemakers. Contact Dermatitis 34:17–22

179. Diphenylthiourea

CAS Registry Number [102–08–9]

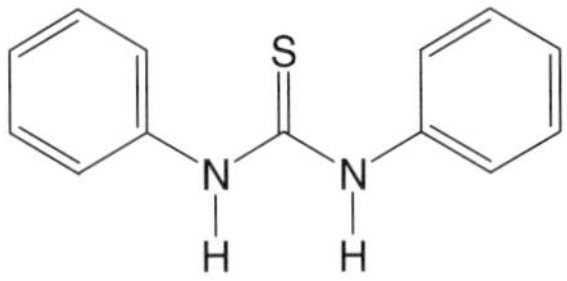

It is a rubber chemical used as an accelerator and stabilizing agent in neoprene.

Suggested Reading

Kanerva L, Estlander T, Jolanki R (1994) Occupational allergic contact dermatitis caused by thiourea compounds. Contact Dermatitis 31: 242–248

Kiec-Swierczynska M (1995) Occupational sensitivity to rubber. Contact Dermatitis 32:171–172

180. Disperse Blue 106

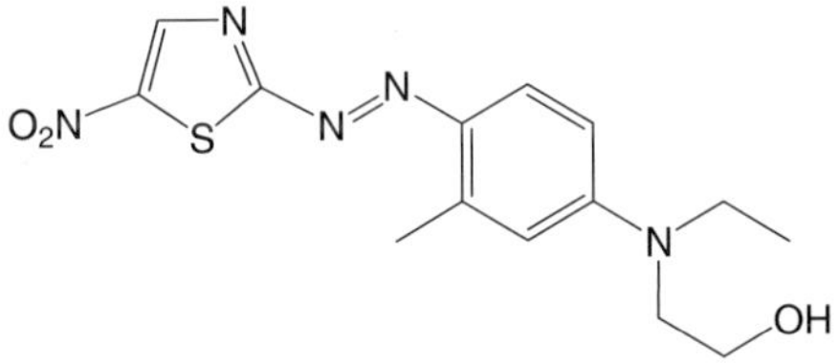

This clothing dye used in synthetic fibers is one of the most potent sensitizers in clothes. Allergic contact dermatitis is relatively frequent in consumers. Occupational textile dye dermatitis was reported in a ready-to-wear shop. Constant concomitant reactions with Disperse Blue 124 are due to their chemical similarities, as with photograph developers CD1, CD2, CD3, and CD4.

Suggested Reading

Menezes-Brandão F, Altermatt C, Pecegueiro M, Bordalo O, Foussereau J (1985) Contact dermatitis to Disperse Blue 106. Contact Dermatitis 13: 80–84

Mota F, Silva E, Varela P, Azenha A, Massa A (2000) An outbreak of occupational textile dye dermatitis from Disperse Blue 106. Contact Dermatitis 43:235–236

181. Disperse Blue 124

CAS Registry Number [15141–18–1]

This clothing dye used in synthetic fibers is one of the most potent sensitizers in clothes. It is a textile dye responsible for occupational contact dermatitis in the textile industry. A positive patch test reaction was observed in a painter sensitized to phthalocyanine dyes, with no occupational relevance. Constant concomitant reactions with Disperse Blue 106, and even to photographic developers CD1–4, are due to their chemical similarities.

Suggested Reading
Raccagni AA, Baldari U, Righini MG (1996) Airborne dermatitis in a painter. Contact Dermatitis 35 : 119–120
Soni BP, Sherertz EF (1996) Contact dermatitis in the textile industry: a review of 72 patients. Am J Contact Dermat 7 : 226–230

182. Disperse Dyes

Disperse dyes are so-called because they are partially soluble in water. These synthetic dyes have either an anthraquinone (disperse anthraquinone dyes) or an azoic structure (disperse azo dyes). They are the most commonly employed dyes, sometimes as hair dyes, but chiefly in the textile industry to color synthetic fibers such as polyester, acrylic and acetate, and sometimes nylon, particularly in stockings. They are not used for natural fibers. These molecules are the main textile sensitizers.

183. Disperse Orange 3

CI 11005

CAS Registry Number [730–40–5]

Disperse Orange 3 is an azo dye that can induce contact dermatitis in workers in the textile industry. It is positive in a great majority of PPD-positive people, because of hydrolysis in the skin into PPD. Disperse Orange 3 can also be found in some semipermanent hair dyes.

Suggested Reading

Balato N, Lembo G, Patruno C, Ayala F (1990) Prevalence of textile dye contact sensitization. Contact Dermatitis 23:126–127

Condé-Salazar L, Baz M, Guimaraens D, Cannavo A (1995) Contact dermatitis in hairdressers: patch test results in 379 hairdressers (1980–1993). Am J Contact Dermat 6:19–23

Soni BP, Sherertz EF (1996) Contact dermatitis in the textile industry: a review of 72 patients. Am J Contact Dermat 7:226–230

184. Disperse Orange 31

CAS Registry Number [61968-38-5] (and [68391-42-4]?)

The synthetic azo dye Disperse Orange 31 was wrongly substituted by Disperse Orange 3 in patch test materials from Chemotechnique. This situation explains why a relatively low percentage of patients positive to PPD were positive to Disperse Orange 3, although a co-reaction is explained to be very frequent because skin transformation of Disperse Orange 3 into PPD.

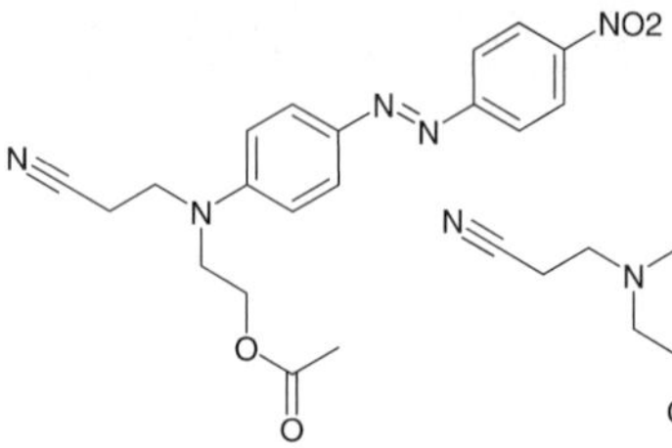

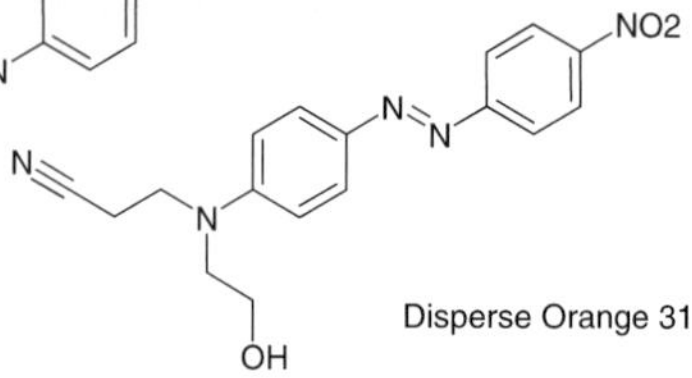

Disperse Orange 31 hydrolyzed

Disperse Orange 31

Suggested Reading

Goon AT, Gilmour NJ, Basketter DA, White IR, Rycroft RJ, McFadden JP
(2003) High frequency of simultaneous sensitivity to Disperse Orange
3 in patients with positive patch tests to para-phenylenediamine. Contact Dermatitis 48:248–250

Le Coz CJ, Jelen G, Goossens A, Vigan M, Ducombs G, Bircher A, Giordano-
Labadie F, Pons-Guiraud A, Milpied-Homsi B, Castelain M, Tennstedt
D, Bourrain JL, Bernard G, GERDA (2004) Disperse (yes), Orange
(yes), 3 (no): what do we test in textile dye dermatitis? Contact Dermatitis 50:126–127

185. Disperse Red 11

CI 62015

CAS Registry Number [2872–48–2]

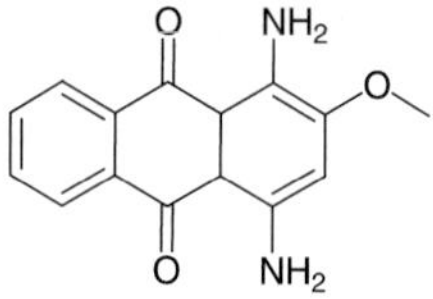

Disperse Red 11 is an example of disperse dye anthraquinone type.

Suggested Reading

Cronin E (1980) Contact dermatitis. Churchill Livingstone, Edinburgh,
pp 36–92

186. Disperse Yellow 3

CI 11855

CAS Registry Number
[2832–40–8]

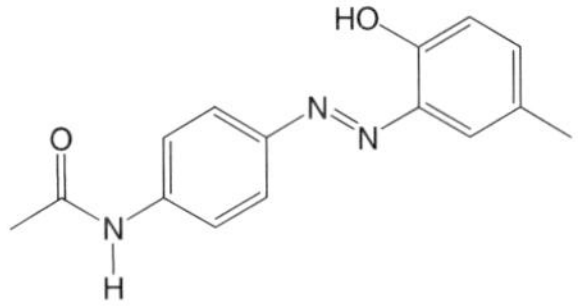

This azoic dye is responsible for textile dermatitis from stockings and occupational contact dermatitis in workers in the textile industry. It can be found in some semipermanent hair dyes.

Suggested Reading

Condé-Salazar L, Baz M, Guimaraens D, Cannavo A (1995) Contact dermatitis in hairdressers: patch test results in 379 hairdressers (1980–1993). Am J Contact Dermat 6:19–23

Soni BP, Sherertz EF (1996) Contact dermatitis in the textile industry: a review of 72 patients. Am J Contact Dermat 7:226–230

187. Dithianone

CAS Registry Number
[3347–22–6]

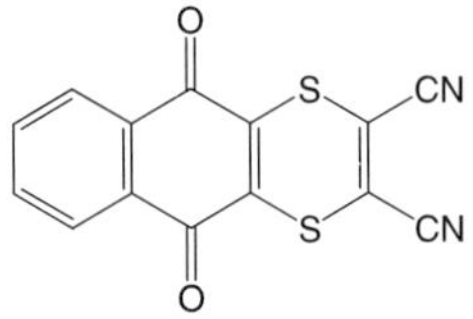

Dithianone is an anthraquinone derivative, used as a fungicide agent. With cymoxanil, it is contained in Aktuan®. Cases in agricultural workers were reported sparsely.

Suggested Reading

Koch P (1996) Occupational allergic contact dermatitis and airborne contact dermatitis from 5 fungicides in a vineyard worker. Cross-reactions between fungicides of the dithiocarbamate group? Contact Dermatitis 34:324–329

188. Dodecyl Gallate

Lauryl Gallate

CAS Registry Number
[1166–52–5]

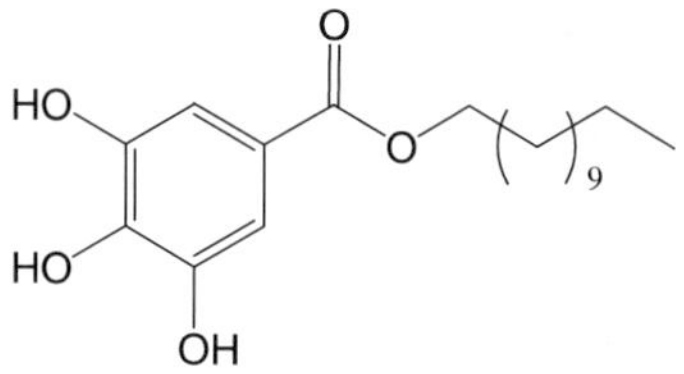

This gallic acid ester (E 310) is an antioxidant added to foods and cosmetics to prevent oxidation of unsaturated fatty acids. Cases were reported in workers of the food industry, gallate being contained in margarine, and from washing powder.

Suggested Reading
De Groot AC, Gerkens F (1990) Occupational airborne contact dermatitis from octyl gallate. Contact Dermatitis 23:184–186
Mancuso G, Staffa M, Errani A, Berdondini RM, Fabri P (1990) Occupational dermatitis in animal feed mill workers. Contact Dermatitis 22:37–41

189. Doxepin

CAS Registry Number [1668–19–5]

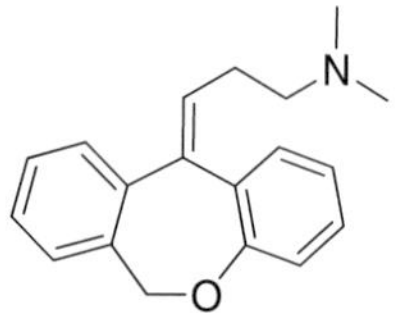

This benzoxepin tricylcic drug has antidepressant, anticholinergic, anti-itching, and antihistamine properties. After oral use, it has been developed as a topical anti-itching agent. Allergic contact dermatitis is not infrequent.

Suggested Reading
Buckley DA (2000) Contact allergy to doxepin. Contact Dermatitis 43:231–232
Taylor JS, Praditsuwan P, Handel D, Kuffner G (1996) Allergic contact dermatitis from doxepin cream. One-year patch test clinic experience. Arch Dermatol 132:515–518

190. Epichlorhydrin

1-Chloro-2,3-Epoxypropane

CAS Registry Number [106–89–8]

Epoxy resin of the Bisphenol A type is synthesized from epichlorhydrin and bisphenol A. It leads to bisphenol A diglycidyl ether, which is the monomer of bisphenol-A-based epoxy resins. Sensitization to epichlorhydrin occurs mainly in workers of the epoxy resin industry. Sensitization in individuals not working at epoxy resin plants is rare. It has however been described to occur following exposure to a soil fumigant, due to solvent cement and in a worker in a pharmaceutical plant, in a division of drug synthesis. Epichlorhydrin was used for the production of drugs propranolol and oxprenolol.

Suggested Reading

Holness DL, Nethercott JR (1993) The performance of specialized collections of bisphenol A epoxy resin system components in the evaluation of workers in an occupational health clinic population. Contact Dermatitis 28 : 216–219

Rebandel P, Rudzki E (1990) Dermatitis caused by epichlorhydrin, oxprenolol hydrochloride and propranolol hydrochloride. Contact Dermatitis 23 : 199

Van Jost T, Roesyanto ID, Satyawan I (1990) Occupational sensitization to epichlorhydrin (ECH) and bisphenol-A during the manufacture of epoxy resin. Contact Dermatitis 22 : 125–126

191. Epoxy Resins of the Bisphenol A Type

These resins are synthesized from bisphenol A and epichlorhydrin. Hardeners are added, such as amines (ethylenediamine, diethylenetriamine, triethylenetetramine, isophoronediamine, triethylenetriamine and 4,4'-diaminophenylmethane) or acid anhydrides (phthalic anhydride). Reactive diluents may be added, such as allyl glycidyl ether, butanediol diglycidyl ether, *n*-butyl glycidyl ether, *o*-cresyl glycidyl ether, hexanediol diglycidyl ether, neopentyl glycol diglycidyl ether, phenyl glycidyl ether, glycidyl ester of synthetic fatty acids, and glycidyl ether of aliphatic alcohols (Epoxide-8).

Suggested Reading

Holness DL, Nethercott JR (1993) The performance of specialized collections of bisphenol A epoxy resin system components in the evaluation of workers in an occupational health clinic population. Contact Dermatitis 28 : 216–219

Jolanki R, Kanerva L, Estlander T, Tarvainen K, Keskinen H, Henriks-Eckerman ML (1990) Occupational dermatoses from epoxy resin compounds. Contact Dermatitis 23 : 172–183

192. 2,3-Epoxypropyl Trimethyl Ammonium Chloride

EPTMAC, Glycidyl Trimethyl Ammonium Chloride, Oxiranemethanaminium, *N,N, N*-Trimethyl Chloride

CAS Registry Number [3033–77–0]

Used in the production of cationic starch for the paper industry, EPTMAC caused contact dermatitis in workers.

Suggested Reading

Estlander T, Jolanki R, Kanerva L (1997) Occupational allergic contact dermatitis from 2,3-epoxypropyl trimethyl ammonium chloride (EPTMAC) and Kathon R LX in a starch modification factory. Contact Dermatitis 36 : 191–194

193. Estradiol

17-β-Estradiol, (17β)-Estra-1,3,5(10)-Triene-3,17-diol

CAS Registry Number [50–28–2]

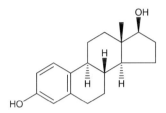

Natural estradiol, used in transdermal systems for hormonal substitution, can induce allergic contact dermatitis, with the risk of systemic contact dermatitis after oral reintroduction.

Suggested Reading

Gonçalo M, Oliveira HS, Monteiro C, Clerins I, Figueiredo A (1999) Allergic and systemic contact dermatitis from estradiol. Contact Dermatitis 40:58–59

194. Ethoxyquin

1,2-Dihydro 6-Ethoxy 2,2,4-Trimethylquinolein, Santoquin®, Santoflex®

CAS Registry Number [91–53–2]

Ethoxyquin is used as an antioxidant in animal feed and caused contact dermatitis in a worker at an animal feed mill.

Suggested Reading

Mancuso G, Staffa M, Errani A, Berdondini RM, Fabri P (1990) Occupational dermatitis in animal feed mill workers. Contact Dermatitis 22: 37–41

195. Ethyl Alcohol

Ethanol

CAS Registry Number [64–17–5]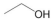

Ethanol is widely used for its solvent and antiseptic properties. It is rather an irritant and sensitization has rarely been reported.

Suggested Reading
Ophaswongse S, Maibach HI (1994) Alcohol dermatitis: allergic contact dermatitis and contact urticaria syndrome. Contact Dermatitis 30 : 1–6
Patruno C, Suppa F, Sarraco G, Balato N (1994) Allergic contact dermatitis due to ethyl alcohol. Contact Dermatitis 31 : 124

196. 4-Ethyl-Pyridine

CAS Registry Number [536–75–4]

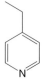

4-Ethyl-pyridine is used as a monomer in polymer chemistry.

Suggested Reading
Sasseville D, Balbul A, Kwong P, Yu K (1996) Contact sensitization to pyridine derivatives. Contact Dermatitis 35 : 101–102

197. Ethylbutylthiourea

CAS Registry Number [32900–06–4]

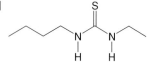

Ethylbutylthiourea is an accelerator used with other thiourea derivatives in the production of neoprene rubber. It is also contained in glues, mainly neoprene type.

Suggested Reading

Bergendorff O, Persson CML, Hansson C (2004) HPLC analysis of alkyl thioureas in an orthopaedic brace and patch testing with pure ethylbutylthiourea. Contact Dermatitis 51: 273–277

Kanerva L, Estlander T, Jolanki R (1994) Occupational allergic contact dermatitis caused by thiourea compounds. Contact Dermatitis 31: 242–248

Roberts JL, Hanifin JM (1980) Contact allergy and cross-reactivity to substituted thiourea compounds. Contact Dermatitis 6: 138–139

198. Ethylene Oxide

CAS Registry Number [75–21–8]

Ethylene oxide is a very strong irritant widely used in the chemical industry, and as a sterilizer of medical supplies, pharmaceutical products, and food. Residues in masks or dressings can produce irritant contact dermatitis.

Suggested Reading

Lerman Y, Ribak J, Skulsky M, Ingber A (1995) An outbreak of irritant contact dermatitis from ethylene oxide among pharmaceutical workers. Contact Dermatitis 33: 280–281

199. Ethylenediamine

CAS Registry Number [107–15–3]

Ethylenediamine is used in numerous industrial processes as a solvent for casein or albumin, as a stabilizer in rubber latex and as a textile lubricant. It can be found in epoxy resin hardeners, cooling oils, fungicides, and waxes. Contact dermatitis from ethylenediamine is almost exclusively due to topical medicaments. Occupational contact dermatitis in epoxy resin systems is rather infrequent. Ethylenediamine can cross-react with triethylenetetramine and diethylenetriamine. Ethylenediamine was found to be responsible for sensitization in pharmacists handling aminophylline suppositories, in nurses preparing and administering injectable theophylline, and in a laboratory technician in the manufacture of aminophylline tablets.

Suggested Reading

Chieregato C, Vincenzi C, Guerra L, Farina P (1994) Occupational allergic contact dermatitis due to ethylenediamine dihydrochloride and cresyl glycidyl ether in epoxy resin systems. Contact Dermatitis 30:120

Corazza M, Mantovani L, Trimurti L, Virgili A (1994) Occupational contact sensitization to ethylenediamine in a nurse. Contact Dermatitis 31: 328–329

Jolanki R, Kanerva L, Estlander T, Tarvainen K, Keskinen H, Henriks-Eckerman ML (1990) Occupational dermatoses from epoxy resin compounds. Contact Dermatitis 23:172–183

Mancuso G, Reggiani M, Berdondini RM (1996) Occupational dermatitis in shoemakers. Contact Dermatitis 34:17–22

Sasseville D, Al-Khenaizan S (1997) Occupational contact dermatitis from ethylenediamine in a wire-drawing lubricant. Contact Dermatitis 3: 228–229

200. Ethylenethiourea

CAS Registry Number [96–45–7]

Ethylenethiourea, a thiourea derivative, is a rubber chemical. It caused contact dermatitis mainly in rubber workers.

Suggested Reading

Bruze M, Fregert S (1983) Allergic contact dermatitis from ethylenethiourea. Contact Dermatitis 9:208–212

Kanerva L, Estlander T, Jolanki R (1994) Occupational allergic contact dermatitis caused by thiourea compounds. Contact Dermatitis 31: 242–248

201. Ethylhexylglycerin

Octoxyglycerin

CAS Registry Number [70445–33–9]

This glycerol monoalkylether is used as a skin conditioning agent, with bactericidal properties against Gram-positive bacteria.

Suggested Reading

Linsen G, Goossens A (2002) Allergic contact dermatitis from ethylhexylglycerin. Contact Dermatitis 47:169

202. Eugenol

CAS Registry Number [97–53–0]

Eugenol is a fragrance allergen obtained from many natural sources. Occupational sensitization to eugenol may occur in dental profession workers. Eugenol is contained in "fragrance mix" and has to be listed by name in cosmetics within the EU.

Suggested Reading

Berova N, Stranky L, Krasteva M (1990) Studies on contact dermatitis in stomatological staff. Dermatol Monatsschr 176:15–18

Rudzki E, Rebandel P, Grzywa Z (1989) Patch tests with occupational contactants in nurses, doctors and dentists. Contact Dermatitis 20:247–250

203. Euxyl®K 400 (see 284. subentry 1,2-Dibromo-2,4-Dicyanobutane and 322. Phenoxyethanol)

Euxyl®K 400 is a mixture of 1,2-dibromo-2,4-dicyanobutane 20% and phenoxyethanol 80%, widely utilized as a preservative in cosmetics, hand creams and toiletries, but also in water-based paints, glues, metalworking fluids, and detergents. Sensitization was reported in masseurs, in a beautician, an offset printer, and a hospital cleaner. We observed four cases of hand contact dermatitis in metalworkers, due to the so-called Euxyl® K 400 contained in barrier creams. No sensitization was observed to phenoxyethanol (personal cases).

Suggested Reading

Aalto-Korte K, Jolanki R, Estlander T, Alanko K, Kanerva L (1996) Occupational allergic contact dermatitis caused by Euxyl K 400. Contact Dermatitis 35:193–194

204. Famotidine

CAS Registry Number [76824–35–6]

Contact dermatitis in a nurse from famotidine, an H_2-receptor agonist, was described. In industry, three cases were reported due to intermediates of the synthesis of 2-diamino-ethylene-amino-thiazolyl-methylenethiourea-dichloride, and 4-chloromethyl-2-guanidinothiazole-nitrochloride.

Suggested Reading

Guimaraens D, Gonzales MA, Condé-Salazar L (1994) Occupational allergic contact dermatitis from intermediate products in famotidine synthesis. Contact Dermatitis 31:259–260

Monteseirin J, Conde J (1990) Contact eczema from famotidine. Contact Dermatitis 22:290

205. Farnesol

3,7,11-Trimethyldodeca-2,6,10-Trienol (Four Isomers)

CAS Registry Numbers [4602–84–0] for the mixture, [106–28–5] for the *trans/trans*, [3790–71–4] for the *cis/trans*, [3879–60–5] for the *trans/cis*, and [16106–95–9] for the *cis/cis*

Farnesol is one of the most frequent contact allergens in perfumes. It is contained in small amounts in *Myroxylon pereirae* and in poplar buds. It is a blend of four diastereosiomers *trans/cis*.

As a fragrance allergen, farnesol has to be mentioned by name in cosmetics within the EU.

Suggested Reading

Frosch PJ, Johansen JD, Menné T, Pirker C, Rastogi SC, Andersen KE, Bruze M, Goossens A, Lepoittevin JP, White IR (2002) Further important sensitizers in patients sensitive to fragrances. Contact Dermatitis 47: 78–85

Schnuch A, Uter W, Geier J, Lessmann H, Frosch PJ (2004) Contact allergy to farnesol in 2021 consecutively patch tested patients. Results of the IVDK. Contact Dermatitis 50:117–121

206. Fenvalerate

CAS Registry Number [51630–58–1]

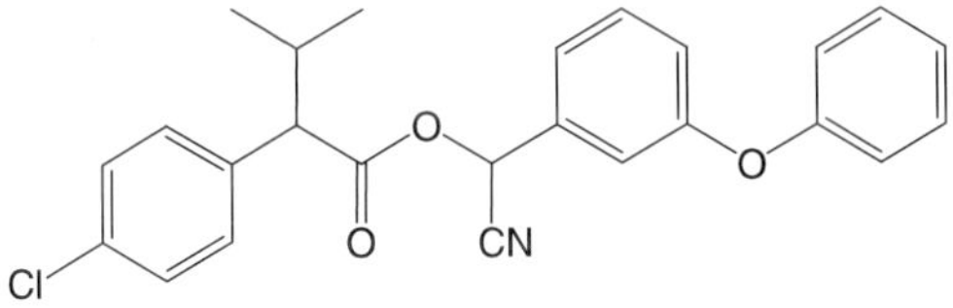

Fenvalerate is an insecticide of the synthetic pyrethroid group, which induced sensitization in farmers.

Suggested Reading

Sharma VK, Kaur S (1990) Contact sensitization by pesticides in farmers. Contact Dermatitis 23:77–80

207. Fluazinam

Shirlan®, 3-Chloro-N-(3-Chloro-5-Trifluoromethyl-2-Pyridyl)-Trifluoro-2,6-Dinitro-p-Toluidine

CAS Registry Number [79622–59–6]

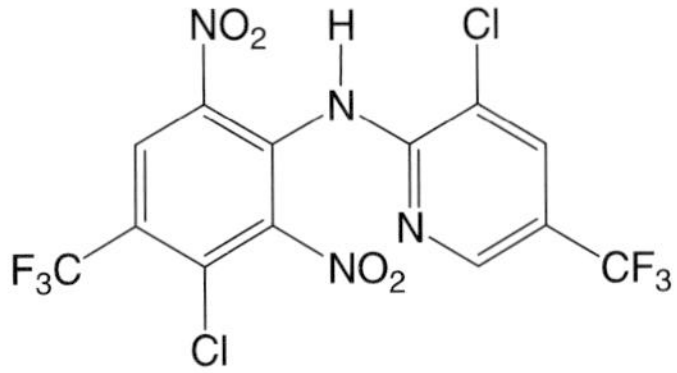

Fluazinam is a pesticide with a broad spectrum of antifungal activity. It caused sensitization in employees in the tulip bulb industry and in farmers. Fluazinam induced contact dermatitis in a worker in a plant where it was manufactured.

Suggested Reading

Bruynzeel DP, Tafelkruijer J, Wilks MF (1995) Contact dermatitis due to a new fungicide used in the tulip bulb industry. Contact Dermatitis 33: 8–11

Van Ginkel CJW, Sabapathy NN (1995) Allergic contact dermatitis from the newly introduced fungicide fluazinam. Contact Dermatitis 32: 160–162

208. Flutamide

2-Methyl-*N*-[4-Nitro-3-(Trifluoromethyl)Phenyl]Propan-amide,
Trifluoro-2-Methyl-4′-Nitro-*m*-Propionotoluidide,
4′-Nitro-3′-Trifluoromethylisobutyranilide, Niftolid

CAS Registry Number [13311–84–7]

Flutamide is an anti-androgenic hormonal anti-neoplastic drug that can induce photosensitivity and porphyria-like eruption.

Suggested Reading

Borroni G, Brazzelli V, Baldini F, Borghini F, Gaviglio MR, Beltrami B, Nolli G (1998) Flutamide-induced pseudoporphyria. Br J Dermatol 138:711–712

Martín-Lázaro J, Goday Buján J, Parra Arrondo A, Rodríguez Lozano J, Cuerda Galindo E, Fonseca Capdevila E (2004) Is photopatch testing useful in the investigation of photosensitivity due to flutamide? Contact Dermatitis 50:325–326

209. Folpet

Folpel, Phthalane, Trichloromethylthiophthalimide

CAS Registry Number [133-07-3]

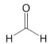

Folpet is a pesticide, fungicide agent of thiophthalimide group. Occupational exposure occurs mostly in agricultural workers or in florists. Photosensitivity has been reported.

Suggested Reading

Lisi P, Caraffini S, Assalve D (1987) Irritation and sensitization potential of pesticides. Contact Dermatitis 17 : 212–218

Mark KA, Brancaccio RR, Soter NA, Cohen DE (1999) Allergic contact and photoallergic contact dermatitis to plant and pesticide allergens. Arch Dermatol 135 : 67–70

Peluso AM, Tardio M, Adamo F, Venturo N (1991) Multiple sensitization due to bis-dithiocarbamate and thiophthalimide pesticides. Contact Dermatitis 25 : 327

210. Formaldehyde

Methanal, Formalin

CAS Registry Number [50-00-0]

Sources and uses of formaldehyde are numerous. Exposed people are mainly health workers, cleaners, painters, metalworkers, but also photographers (color developers) and carbonless copy paper users. Formaldehyde can induce contact urticaria. Formaldehyde may be the cause of sensitization to formaldehyde releasers: benzyl-hemiformal, bromonitrodioxane, bromonitropropanediol (?), chloroallylhexaminium chloride or Quaternium-15, diazolidinyl-urea, dimethylol urea, dimethyloldimethylhydantoin or DMDM hydantoin, hexamethylenetetramine or methenamine, imidazoli-dinylurea, monomethyloldimethylhydantoin or MDM hydantoin, N-methylolchloracetamide, paraformaldehyde and trihydroxy-ethylhexahydrotriazine or Grotan BK.

Formaldehyde is used for the synthesis of many resins. Some of them, such as formaldehyde-urea and melamine-formaldehyde resins, can be used in textiles and secondarily release free formaldehyde).

Other resins, such as *p-tert*-butyl-phenol formaldehyde resin or tosylamine formaldehyde resin, do not release formaldehyde.

Suggested Reading

Flyvholm MA, Menné T (1992) Allergic contact dermatitis from formaldehyde. A case study focussing on sources of formaldehyde exposure. Contact Dermatitis 27:27–36

Murray R (1991) Health aspects of carbonless copy paper. Contact Dermatitis 24:321–333

Pabst R (1987) Exposure to formaldehyde in anatomy: an occupational health hazard? Anat Rec 219:109–112

Rudzki E, Rebandel P, Grzywa Z (1989) Patch tests with occupational contactants in nurses, doctors and dentists. Contact Dermatitis 20:247–250

Scheman AJ, Katta R (1997) Photographic allergens: an update. Contact Dermatitis 37:130

Torresani C, Periti I, Beski L (1996) Contact urticaria syndrome from formaldehyde with multiple physical urticaria. Contact Dermatitis 35:174–175

---

211. Frullanolide

L(–) Frullanolide

CAS Registry Number [27579–97–1]

D(+) Frullanolide

CAS Registry Number [40776–40–7]

Frullanolide is a sesquiterpene lactone, contained in *Frullania tamarisci* Dum. (L-Frullanolide) and *Frullania dilatata* Dum. (Dfrullanolide), a lichen that grows on lobed-leaf trees such as oak and beech. Sensitivity causes airborne and sometimes severe polymorphous erythema-like allergic contact dermatitis, mainly in foresters and in people using firewood, lumbermen, sawyers, carpenters, and merchants in rough timber.

Suggested Reading

Ducombs G, Lepoittevin JP, Berl V, Andersen KE, Brandão FM, Bruynzeel DP, Bruze M, Camarasa JG, Frosch PJ, Goossens A, Lachapelle JM, Lahti A, Le Coz CJ, Maibach HI, Menné T, Seidenari S, Shaw S, Tosti A, Wilkinson JD (2003) Routine patch testing with frullanolide mix: an European Environmental and Contact Dermatitis Research Group multicentre study. Contact Dermatitis 48:158–161

Quirino AP, Barros MA (1995) Occupational contact dermatitis from lichens and *Frullania*. Contact Dermatitis 33:68–69

Tomb RR (1992) Patch testing with frullania during a 10-year period: hazards and complications. Contact Dermatitis 26:220–223

212. Furaltadone

5-Morpholinomethyl-3 (5-Nitrofurfurilidenamine)-2-Oxazolidinone

CAS Registry Number [139–91–3]

This nitrofuran derivative can be added in animal feed or in eardrops.

Suggested Reading

Sánchez-Pérez J, Córdoba S, Jesús del Río M, García-Díes A (1999) Allergic contact dermatitis from furaltadone in eardrops. Contact Dermatitis 40:222

Vilaplana J, Grimalt F, Romaguera C (1990) Contact dermatitis from furaltadone in animal feed. Contact Dermatitis 22:232–233

213. Furazolidone

3-(5-Nitrofurfurylideneamino)-2-Oxazolidinone

CAS Registry Number
[67–45–8]

Furazolidone belongs to the group of nitrofurans. This antimicrobial (antibacterial and antiprotozoal) agent is used in veterinary medicine both topically and orally, particularly in animal feed. Reactions are reported in workers exposed to it in animal feeds. Cross-reactions with other nitrofuran derivatives are rare.

Suggested Reading

Burge S, Bransbury A (1994) Allergic contact dermatitis due to furazolidone in a piglet medication. Contact Dermatitis 31:199–200

De Groot AC, Conemans MH (1990) Contact allergy to furazolidone. Contact Dermatitis 22:202–205

214. Geraniol

3,7-Dimethyl-2,6-Octadien-1-ol

CAS Registry Number [106–24–1]

cis-Geraniol: Nerol

CAS Registry Number [106–25–2]

trans-Geraniol: Citrol

CAS Registry Number [624–15–7]

Geraniol is an olefinic terpene, constituting the chief part of rose oil and oil of palmarosa. It is also found in many other essential oils such as citronella, lemon grass or ylang-ylang (*Cananga odorata* Hook.f. and Thoms.). It is contained in most fine fragrances and in "fragrance mix." As a fragrance allergen, geraniol has to be mentioned by name in cosmetics within the EU.

Suggested Reading

Frosch PJ, Johansen JD, Menné T, Pirker C, Rastogi SC, Andersen KE, Bruze M, Goossens A, Lepoittevin JP, White IR (2002) Further important sensitizers in patients sensitive to fragrances. Contact Dermatitis 47: 78–85

Kanerva L, Estlander T, Jolanki R (1995) Occupational allergic contact dermatitis caused by ylang-ylang oil. Contact Dermatitis 33:198–199

215. Glutaraldehyde

Glutaral, Pentanedial, Glutaric Dialdehyde

CAS Registry Number [111–30–8]

Glutaraldehyde is a well-know sensitizer in cleaners and health workers. It can also be found in X-ray developers or in cosmetics.

Suggested Reading

Cusano F, Luciano S (1993) Contact allergy to benzalkonium chloride and glutaraldehyde in a dental nurse. Contact Dermatitis 28:127

Nethercott JR, Holness DL, Page E (1988) Occupational contact dermatitis due to glutaraldehyde in health care workers. Contact Dermatitis 18: 193–196

Scheman AJ, Katta R (1997) Photographic allergens: an update. Contact Dermatitis 37:130

Stingeni L, Lapomarda V, Lisi P (1995) Occupational hand dermatitis in hospital environments. Contact Dermatitis 33:172–176

Taylor JS, Praditsuwan P (1996) Latex allergy. Review of 44 cases including outcome and frequent association with allergic hand eczema. Arch Dermatol 32:265–271

216. Glyceryl Thioglycolate

Glyceryl Monothioglycolate, Glycerol Monomercaptoacetate

CAS Registry Number [30618–84–9]

It is an acid permanent-wave ingredient, which induces contact dermatitis in hairdressers.

Suggested Reading

Frosch PJ, Burrows D, Camarasa JG, Dooms-Goossens A, Ducombs G, Lahti A, Menné T, Rycroft RJG, Shaw S, White IR, Wilkinson JD (1993) Allergic reactions to a hairdresser's series: results from 9 European centres. Contact Dermatitis 28:180–183

Guerra L, Tosti A, Bardazzi F, Pigatto P, Lisi P, Santucci B, Valsecchi R, Schena D, Angelini G, Sertoli A, Ayala F, Kokelj F (1992) Contact dermatitis in hairdressers: the Italian experience. Gruppo Italiano Ricerca Dermatiti da Contatto e Ambientali. Contact Dermatitis 26:101–107

Van der Walle HB, Brunsveld VM (1994) Dermatitis in hairdressers (I). The experience of the past 4 years. Contact Dermatitis 30:217–220

217. Glycidyl 1-Naphthyl Ether

1-Naphthyl-Glycidyl Ether

CAS Registry Number [2461–42–9]

Glycidyl ethers are used as reactive diluents for epoxy resins. Alpha-naphthyl glycidyl ether is formed by adding epichlorhydrin and NaOH to alpha-naphthol. Contact dermatitis was reported in workers of a chemical plant.

Suggested Reading

De Groot AC (1994) Occupational contact allergy to alpha-naphthyl glycidyl ether. Contact Dermatitis 30:253–254

218. 3-Glycidyloxypropyltrimethoxysilane

Gamma-Glycidoxypropyltrimethoxysilane, {[(3-(Trimethoxysilyl)Propoxy]methyl}Oxirane

CAS Registry Numbers [2530–83–8], [108727–79–3], [120026–01–9], [138590–36–0] [163035–07–2], [26348–10–7], [51938–40–0], [53029–18–8], [65323–93–5], [88385–40–4]

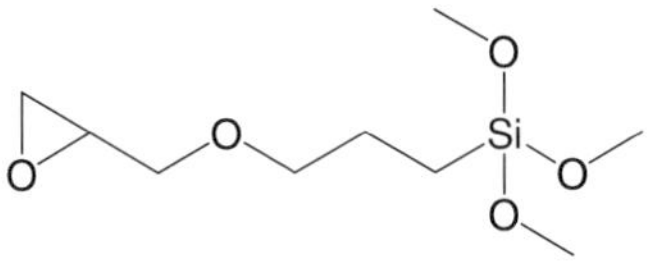

An impurity such as allyl glycidyl ether seemed to be the sensitizing agent contained in 3-glycidyloxypropyltrimethoxysilane.

Suggested Reading

Dooms-Goossens A, Bruze M, Buysse L, Fregert S, Gruvberger B, Stals H (1995) Contact allergy to allyl glycidyl ether present as an impurity in 3-glycidyloxypropyltrimethoxysilane, a fixing additive in silicone and polyurethane. Contact Dermatitis 33:17–19

219. Grotan BK

Hexahydro-1,3,5-Tris-(2-Hydroxyethyl)Triazine

CAS Registry Number [4719–04–4]

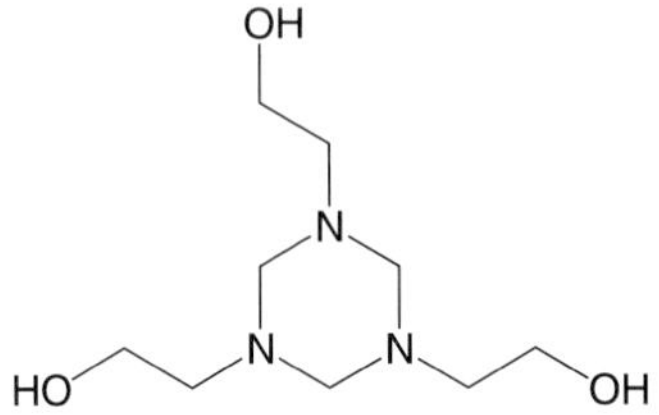

Grotan BK is a triazine derivative contained as a biocide in cutting fluids. It is a formaldehyde releaser. Dermatitis, delayed-type allergic conjunctivitis, and asthma were described.

Suggested Reading

Rasschaert V, Goossens A (2002) Conjunctivitis and bronchial asthma: symptoms of contact allergy to 1,3,5-tris (2-hydroxyethyl)-hexahydrotriazine (Grotan BK). Contact Dermatitis 47:116

Veronesi S, Guerra L, Valeri F, Toni F (1987) Three cases of contact dermatitis sensitive to Grotan BK. Contact Dermatitis 17:255

220. HC Yellow No. 7

Hair Color Yellow No. 7

CAS Registry Number
[104226-21-3]

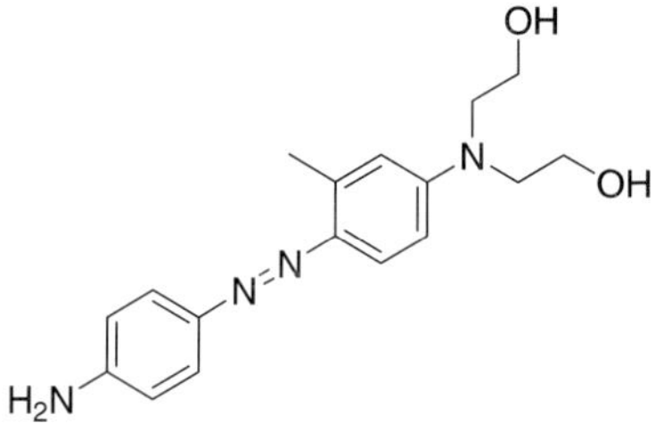

HC Yellow no. 7 is a direct azo dye used in semi-permanent hair dye preparation. Since this dye leads to PPD after hydrolysis, it explains the allergic reaction in PPD-positive patients.

Suggested Reading
Sánchez-Pérez J, García del Río I, Alvares Ruiz S, García Diez A (2004) Allergic contact dermatitis from direct dyes for hair coloration in hairdressers' clients. Contact Dermatitis 50 : 261–262

221. Hexamethylene Diisocyanate

1,6-Hexamethylene Diisocyanate, HDI, HMDI

CAS Registry Number
[822-06-0]

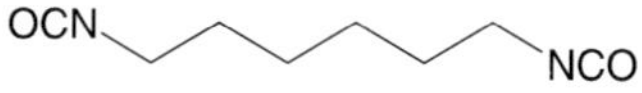

This diisocyanate compound is used in the manufacture of various polyurethane products: elastic and rigid foams, paints, lacquers, adhesives, binding agents, synthetics rubbers, and elastomer fibers.

Suggested Reading
Estlander T, Keskinen H, Jolanki R, Kanerva L (1992) Occupational dermatitis from exposure to polyurethane chemicals. Contact Dermatitis 27 : 161–165

222. Hexamethylenediamine

1,6-Diaminohexane

CAS Registry Number [124–09–4]

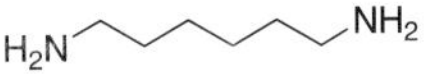

H_2N ⌁ NH_2

Hexamethylenediamine is used with adipic acid in the synthesis of polyamide plastics.

Suggested Reading

Michel PJ, Prost J (1954) Lésions provoquées par l'hexaméthylènediamine. Bull Soc Fr Dermatol Syphiligr 61:385

223. Hexamidine

CAS Registry Number [3811–75–4]

Hexamidine Diisethionate

CAS Registry Number [659–40–5]

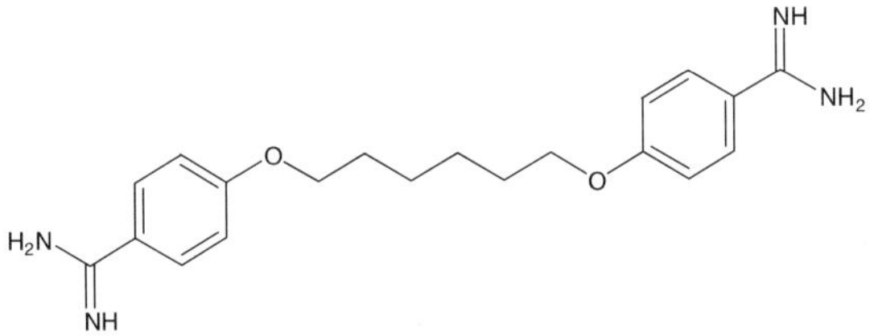

Hexamidine is an antiseptic active against Gram-positive bacteria and fungi, used as a disinfectant and a preservative in cosmetics. It induces papulo-vesicular and diffuse allergic contact dermatitis.

Suggested Reading

Dooms-Goossens A, Vandaele M, Bedert R, Marien K (1989) Hexamidine isethionate: a sensitizer in topical pharmaceutical products and cosmetics. Contact Dermatitis 21:270

Le Coz CJ, Scrivener Y, Santinelli F, Heid E (1998) Sensibilisation de contact au cours des ulcères de jambe. Ann Dermatol Venereol 125:694–699

Revuz J, Poli F, Wechsler J, Dubertret L (1984) Dermatites de contact à l'hexamidine. Ann Dermatol Venereol 111:805–810

224. Hexanediol Diglycidyl Ether

1,6-Hexanediol Diglycidyl Ether

CAS Registry Number [16096–31–4]

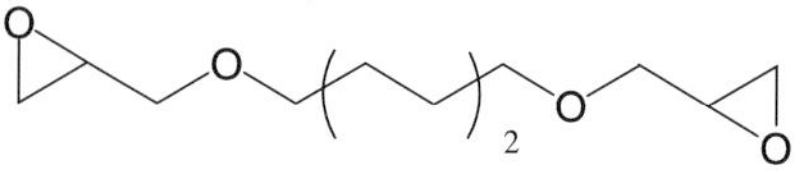

This chemical is a reactive diluent in epoxy resins.

Suggested Reading

Jolanki R, Kanerva L, Estlander T, Tarvainen K, Keskinen H, Henriks-Eckerman ML (1990) Occupational dermatoses from epoxy resin compounds. Contact Dermatitis 23:172–183

225. Hexyl Cinnamic Aldehyde

Hexyl Cinnamaldehyde, Alpha-Hexyl-Cinnamaldehyde, 2-(Phenylmethylene)Octanal, 2-Benzylideneoctanal

CAS Registry Number [101–86–0]

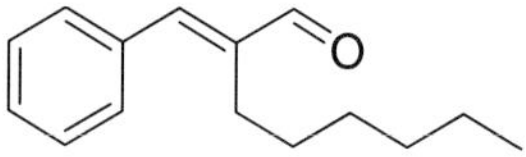

Hexyl cinnamic aldehyde is a fragrance allergen. Its presence has to be mentioned by name in cosmetics within the EU.

Suggested Reading

Frosch PJ, Johansen JD, Menné T, Pirker C, Rastogi SC, Andersen KE, Bruze M, Goossens A, Lepoittevin JP, White IR (2002) Further important sensitizers in patients sensitive to fragrances. Contact Dermatitis 47:78–85

Rastogi SC, Johansen JD, Menné T (1996) Natural ingredients based cosmetics. Content of selected fragrance sensitizers. Contact Dermatitis 34:423–426

226. Hydralazine

CAS Registry Number [86–54–4]

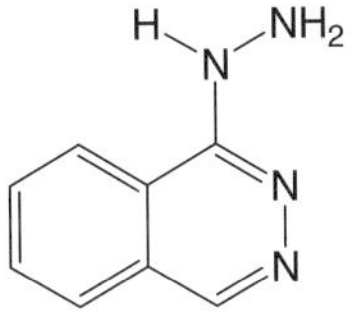

Hydralazine Hydrochloride

CAS Registry Number [304–20–1]

Hydralazine is a hydrazine derivative used as a antihypertensive drug. Skin rashes have been described during treatment. Exposure occurs mainly in the pharmaceutical industry. Cross-sensitivity is frequent with hydrazine, which is considered to be a potent sensitizer.

Suggested Reading

Pereira F, Dias M, Pacheco FA (1996) Occupational contact dermatitis from propranolol, hydralazine, and bendroflumethiazide. Contact Dermatitis 35:303–304

227. Hydrangenol

CAS Registry Number [480–47–7]

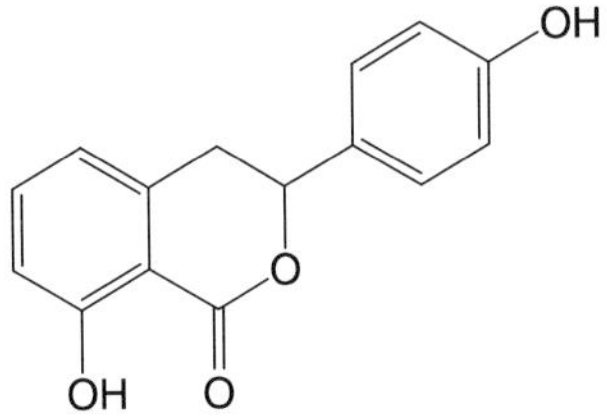

Hydrangenol is the allergen of hydrangea (*Hydrangea macrophylla* Thunb, Hydrangeaceae family).

Suggested Reading

Avenel-Audran M, Hausen BM, Le Sellin J, Ledieu G, Verret JL (2000) Allergic contact dermatitis from hydrangea – is it so rare? Contact Dermatitis 43:189–191

Kuligowski ME, Chang A, Leemreize JHM (1992) Allergic contact hand dermatitis from hydrangea: report of a 10th case. Contact Dermatitis 26:269–270

228. Hydrazine

CAS Registry Number [302–01–2] H_2N—NH_2

Hydrazine sulphate CAS Registry Number [10034–93–2], dihydro-
bromide CAS Registry Number [23268–00–0] and hydrochloride
{14011–37–1] have been reported as occupational sensitizers,
mainly in soldering flux.

Suggested Reading

Frost J, Hjorth N (1959) Contact dermatitis from hydrazine bromide in
     soldering flux. Acta Derm Venereol (Stockh) 39:82–85
Goh CL, Ng SK (1987) Airborne contact dermatitis to colophony in solder-
     ing flux. Contact Dermatitis 17:89–91
Wheeler CE, Penn SR, Cawley EP (1965) Dermatitis from hydrazine hydro-
     bromide solder flux. Arch Dermatol 91:235–239
Wrangsjö K, Martensson A (1986) Hydrazine contact dermatitis from gold
     plating. Contact Dermatitis 15:244–245

229. Hydrocortisone

Cortisol

CAS Registry Number [50–23–7]

Hydrocortisone is the principal glucocorticoid hormone
produced by the adrenal cortex, and is used topically or systemically. It belongs to the allergenic A group. Marker of allergy is
tixocortol pivalate.

Suggested Reading

Lepoittevin JP, Drieghe J, Dooms-Goossens A (1995) Studies in patients with corticosteroid contact allergy. Understanding cross-reactivity among different steroids. Arch Dermatol 131:31–37

Le Coz CJ (2002) Fiche d'éviction en cas d'hypersensibilité au pivalate de tixocortol. Ann Dermatol Venereol 129:348–349

230. Hydrocortisone 17-Butyrate

CAS Registry Number [13609–67–1]

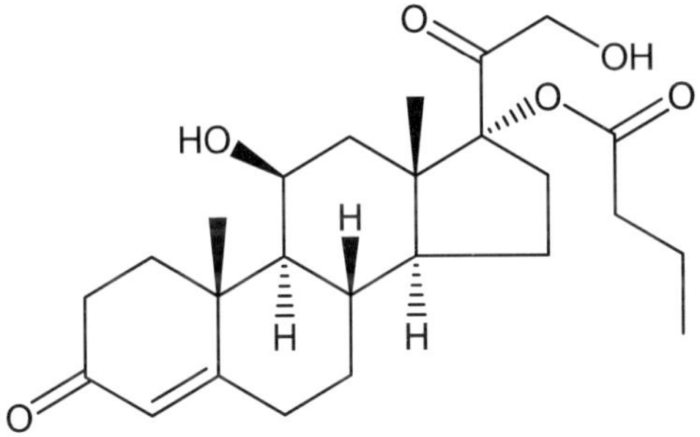

Hydrocortisone 17-butyrate is a C_{17} ester of hydrocortisone. It represents the D2 group of corticosteroids, non C_{16} methylated with a C_{17} ester: hydrocortisone 17-butyrate, hydrocortisone 17-valerate, hydrocortisone aceponate (17-propionate and 21-acetate), methylprednisolone aceponate, and prednicarbate. It is sometimes hydrolyzed in vivo into hydrocortisone, giving allergic reactions to group-A-sensitized people.

Suggested Reading

Le Coz CJ (2002) Fiche d'éviction en cas d'hypersensibilité au 17 butyrate d'hydrocortisone. Ann Dermatol Venereol 129:931

Lepoittevin JP, Drieghe J, Dooms-Goossens A (1995) Studies in patients with corticosteroid contact allergy. Understanding cross-reactivity among different steroids. Arch Dermatol 131:31–37

231. Hydrogen Peroxide

H_2O_2

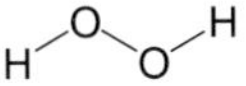

CAS Registry Number [7722–84–1]

Hydrogen peroxide is an oxidizing agent used as a topical antiseptic, and as part of permanent hair-dyes, color-removing preparations, and as a neutralizing agent in permanent waving. The concentration of the hydrogen peroxyde solution is expressed in volume or percentage: 10 volumes correspond to 3%. It is an irritant.

Suggested Reading
Aguirre A, Zabala R, Sanz De Galdeano C, Landa N, Diaz-Perez JL (1994) Positive patch tests to hydrogen peroxide in 2 cases. Contact Dermatitis 30:113

232. Hydroquinone

1,4-Benzenediol

CAS Registry Number [123–31–9]

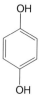

Hydroquinone is used in photography developers (black and white, X-ray, and microfilms), in plastics, in hair dyes as an antioxidant and hair colorant. Hydroquinone is found in many skin bleaching creams.

Suggested Reading
Barrientos N, Ortiz-Frutos J, Gomez E, Iglesias L (2001) Allergic contact dermatitis from a bleaching cream. Am J Contact Dermat 12:33–34

Gebhardt M, Geier J (1996) Evaluation of patch test results with denture material series. Contact Dermatitis 34:191–195

Lidén C, Brehmer-Andersson E (1988) Occupational dermatoses from colour developing agents. Clinical and histopathological observations. Acta Derm Venereol (Stockh) 68:514–522

Scheman AJ, Katta R (1997) Photographic allergens: an update. Contact Dermatitis 37:130

233. (S)-4'-Hydroxy 4-Methoxydalbergione

CAS Registry Number
[3755–63–3]

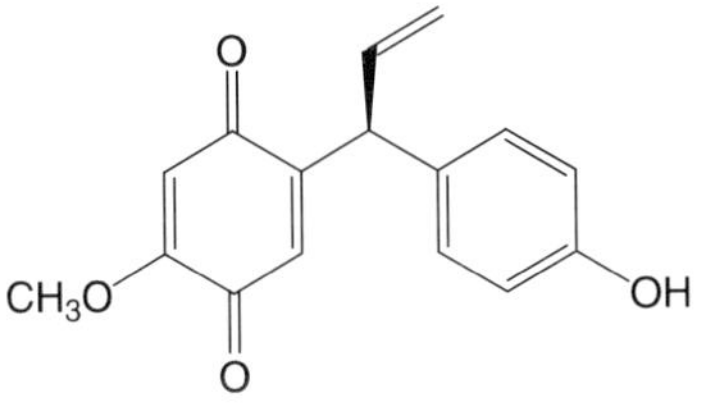

(S)-4'-Hydroxy 4-methoxydalbergione is one of the allergens Brazilian rosewood or Palissander (*Dalbergia nigra* All., Papillionaceae family), cocobolo (*Dalbergia retusa* Hemsl., *Dalbergia granadilla*, and *Dalbergia hypoleuca*) or grenadil (*Dalbergia melanoxylon* Guill. and Perr.).

Suggested Reading
Hausen BM (1981) Wood injurious to human health. A manual. De Gruyter, Berlin

234. Hydroxycitronellal

7-Hydroxycitronellal, Citronellal Hydrate, Laurine, Muguet Synthetic

CAS Registry Number
[107–75–5]

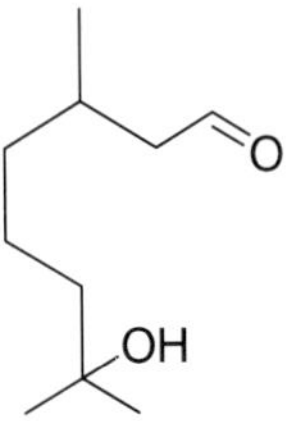

Hydroxycitronellal is a classical fragrance allergen, found in many products. It is contained in "Fragrance Mix." It has to be listed by name in the cosmetics of the EU.

Suggested Reading
Rastogi SC, Johansen JD, Frosch P, Menné T, Bruze M, Lepoittevin JP, Dreier B, Andersen KE, White IR (1998) Deodorants on the European market: quantitative chemical analysis of 21 fragrances. Contact Dermatitis 38:29–35

Svedman C, Bruze M, Johansen JD, Andersen KE, Goossens A, Frosch PJ, Lepoittevin JP, Rastogi S, White IR, Menné T (2003) Deodorants: an experimental provocation study with hydroxycitronellal. Contact Dermatitis 48:217–223

235. Hydroxylamine and Hydroxylammonium Salts

Hydroxylamine

CAS Registry Number [7803–49–8]

Hydroxylammonium Chloride: Hydroxylamine Hydrochloride, Oxammonium Hydrochloride

CAS Registry Numbers [5470–11–1]

Hydroxylammonium Sulfate: Hydroxylamine Sulfate, Oxammonium Sulfate

CAS Registry Number [7803–49–8].

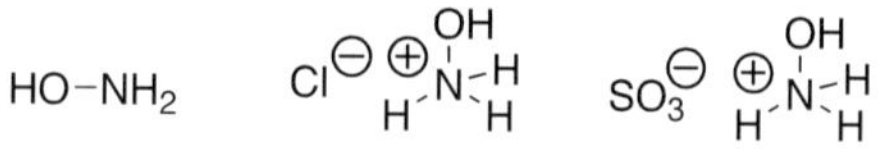

Hydroxylamine and its salts are used in various branches of industry, as reducing agents in color film developers or as reagents in laboratories.

Suggested Reading

Aguirre A, Landa N, Gonzalez M, Diaz-Perez JL (1992) Allergic contact dermatitis in a photographer. Contact Dermatitis 27:340–341
Estlander T, Jolanki T, Kanerva L (1997) Hydroxylammonium chloride as sensitizer in a water laboratory. Contact Dermatitis 36:161–162
Goh CL (1990) Allergic contact dermatitis and onycholysis from hydroxylamine sulphate in colour developer. Contact Dermatitis 22:109

236. Hydroxymethylpentacyclohexenecarboxaldehyde

**Lyral®, Hydroxyisohexyl 3-Cyclohexene Carboxaldehyde,
4-(4-Hydroxy-4-Methylpentyl)-3-Cyclohexene-1-
Carboxaldehyde,
4-(4-Hydroxy-4-Methylpentyl)Cyclohex-3-ene-
Carbaldehyde**

CAS Registry Number [31906–04–4]

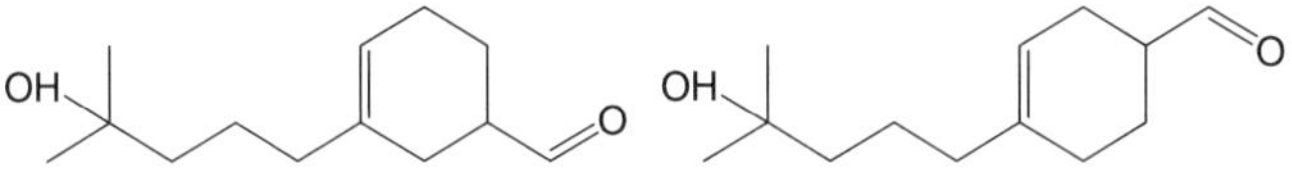

Lyral® is a synthetic blend of two isomers, and one of the most frequently encountered allergen in perfumes. It has to be listed by name in the ingredients of cosmetics in the EU, according to the 7th amendment of the cosmetic directive 76/768/EEC.

Suggested Reading

Johansen JD, Frosch PJ, Svedman C, Andersen KE, Bruze M, Pirker C, Menné T (2003) Hydroxyisohexyl 3-cyclohexene carboxaldehyde – known as Lyral: quantitative aspects and risk assessment of an important fragrance allergen. Contact Dermatitis 48:310–316

237. Hypochlorous Acid and Hypochlorites

Hypochlorous Acid

CAS Registry Number [7790–92–3]

Sodium Hypochlorite

CAS Registry Number [7681–52–9]

Sodium Hypochlorite Hydrate

CAS Registry Number [55248–17–4]

Sodium Hypochlorite Pentahydrate

CAS Registry Number [10022–70–5]

Sodium Hypochlorite Heptahydrate

CAS Registry Number [6431–03–9]

Calcium Hypochlorite

CAS Registry Number [7778–54–3]

Calcium Hypochlorite Dihydroxide

CAS Registry Number [12394–14–8]

Calcium Hypochlorite Dihydrate

CAS Registry Number [22464–76–2]

Calcium Sodium Hypochlorite

CAS Registry Number [53053–57–9]

Lithium Hypochlorite

CAS Registry Number [13840–33–0]

Potassium Hypochlorite

CAS Registry Number [7778–66–7]

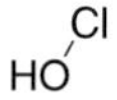

Hypochlorous acid 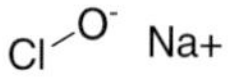   Sodium hypochlorite 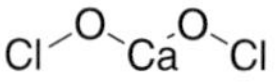   Calcium hypochlorite

Hypochlorites are derived from hypochlorous acid. They are bleaching agents and have large-spectrum antimicrobial activity. Calcium hypochlorite is used for disinfection in swimming pools and in industrial applications and for pulp and textile bleaching. Sodium hypochlorite is used as household laundry bleach, in commercial laundering, in pulp and paper manufacture, in industrial chemical synthesis, and in the disinfection of drinking water. Lithium hypochlorite is used in swimming pools for disinfection and in household detergents. Hypochlorites have caused hand, diffuse or periulcerous dermatitis, due to bleach settings and detergents, swimming pool water, endodontic treatment solution, or ulcer treatment.

Suggested Reading

Salphale PS, Shenoi SD (2003) Contact sensitivity to calcium hypochlorite. Contact Dermatitis 48:162

Sasseville D, Geoffrion CT, Lowry RN (1999) Allergic contact dermatitis from chlorinated swimming pool water. Contact Dermatitis 41: 347–348

238. Imidazolidinyl Urea

Germall® 115, IMIDUREA®

CAS Registry Number [39236–46–9]

Imidazolidinyl urea, a formaldehyde releaser related to diazolidinyl urea (see above), is used as an antimicrobial agent very active against Gram-positive and Gram-negative bacteria, used as a synergist in combination with parabens. It is used as a preservative in aqueous products, mainly in cosmetics, toiletries, and liquid soaps.

Suggested Reading

Karlberg AT, Skare L, Lindberg I, Nyhammar E (1998) A method for quantification of formaldehyde in the presence of formaldehyde donors in skin-care products. Contact Dermatitis 38:20–28

Lachapelle JM, Ale SI, Freeman S, Frosch PJ, Goh CL, Hannuksela M, Hayakawa R, Maibach HI, Wahlberg JE (1997) Proposal for a revised international standard series of patch tests. Contact Dermatitis 36: 121–123

Le Coz CJ (2005) Hypersensibilité à la Diazolidinyl urée et à l'Imidazolidinyl urée. Ann Dermatol Venereol 132:587–588

Van Hecke E, Suys E (1994) Where next to look for formaldehyde? Contact Dermatitis 31:268

239. Iodopropynyl Butylcarbamate

3-Iodo-2-Propynyl-Butyl Carbamate

CAS Registry Number [55406–53–6]

Iodopropynyl butylcarbamate (IPBC) is a broad-spectrum preservative used for years because of its wide field of application, in polymer emulsions and pigment dispersions such as water-based paints and adhesives, cements and inks, as a wood preservative, in metalworking fluids, in household products and in cosmetics. Allergic contact dermatitis to IPBC was reported due to cosmetics, from sanitary wipes, and in metalworkers.

Suggested Reading

Badreshia S, Marks JG Jr (2002) Iodopropynyl butylcarbamate. Am J Contact Dermat 13:77–79

Bryld LE, Agner T, Rastogi SC, Menné T (1997) Iodopropynyl butylcarbamate: a new contact allergen. Contact Dermatitis 36:156–158

Majoie IM, van Ginkel CJW (2000) The biocide iodopropynyl butylcarbamate (IPBC) as an allergen in cutting oils. Contact Dermatitis 43: 238–239

240. Isoeugenol

Isoeugenol

CAS Registry Number [97–54–1]

cis-isoeugenol

CAS Registry Number [5912–86–7]

trans-Isoeugenol

CAS Registry Number [5932–68–3]

Cis-Isoeugenol

Trans-Isoeugenol

Isoeugenol is a mixture of two *cis* and *trans* isomers. It occurs in ylang-ylang and other essential oils. It is a common allergen of perfumes and cosmetics such as deodorants, and is contained in fragrance mix. Its presence in cosmetics is indicated in the INGREDIENTS series. Substitution by esters such as isoeugenyl acetate (not indicated on the package) does not always resolve the allergenic problem, because of the in vivo hydrolysis of the substitute into isoeugenol.

Suggested Reading

Rastogi SC, Johansen JD, Frosch P, Menné T, Bruze M, Lepoittevin JP, Dreier B, Andersen KE, White IR (1998) Deodorants on the European market: quantitative chemical analysis of 21 fragrances. Contact Dermatitis 38:29–35

Tanaka S, Royds C, Buckley D, Basketter DA, Goossens A, Bruze M, Svedman C, Menné T, Johansen JD, White IR, McFadden JP (2004) Contact allergy to isoeugenol and its derivatives: problems with allergen substitution. Contact Dermatitis 51:288–291

241. Alpha-Isomethylionone

3-Buten-2-one, 3-Methyl-4-(2,6,6-Trimethyl-2-Cyclohexen-1-yl), 3-Methyl-4-(2,6,6-Trimethyl-2-Cyclohexen-1-yl)3-Buten-2-one, Cetone Alpha

CAS Registry Number [127–51–5]

As a fragrance allergen, α-isomethylionone has to be mentioned by name in cosmetics within the EU.

Suggested Reading

Frosch PJ (1998) Are major components of fragrances a problem? In: Frosch PJ, Johansen JD, White IR (eds) Fragrances. Beneficial and adverse effects. Springer, Berlin Heidelberg New York, pp 92–99

242. Isophorone Diamine

1-Amino-3-Aminomethyl-3,3,5-Trimethylcyclohexane, 3-Aminomethyl-3,5,5-Trimethylcyclohexylamine

CAS Registry Number [2855–13–2]

Isophorone diamine is widely used in urethane and epoxy coatings for light-stable, weather-resistant properties. It is used in water proofing and paving concreting, and in the manufacture of diisocyanates and polyamides as an epoxy resin hardener. It is a strong sensitizer and can cause airborne contact dermatitis.

Suggested Reading
Guerra L, Vincenzi, Bardazzi F, Tosti A (1992) Contact sensitization to isophoronediamine. Contact Dermatitis 27:52–53

Kelterer D, Bauer A, Elsner P (2000) Spill-induced sensitization to isophorone diamine. Contact Dermatitis 43:110

Lodi A, Mancini LL, Pozzi M, Chiarelli G, Crosti C (1993) Occupational airborne allergic contact dermatitis in parquet layers. Contact Dermatitis 29:281–282

243. Isopropyl Myristate

Tetradecanoic Acid 1-Methyl Ethyl Ester

CAS Registry Number [110–27–0]

Despite wide use in cosmetics, perfumes, and topical medicaments, isopropyl myristate is a very weak sensitizer and a mild irritant.

Suggested Reading
Uter W, Schnuch A, Geier J, Lessmann H (2004) Isopropyl myristate recommended for aimed rather than routine patch testing. Contact Dermatitis 50:242–244

244. *N*-Isopropyl-*N*-Phenyl-4-Phenylenediamine

**IPPD, *N*-Isopropyl-*N*′-Phenyl-*p*-Phenylenediamine,
N-(1-Methylethyl)-*N*′-Phenyl-1,4-Benzenediamine**

CAS Registry Number [101–72–4]

This rubber chemical is used as an antioxidant and anti-ozonant.
The main occupational sources are tires.

Suggested Reading

Condé-Salazar L, Del-Rio E, Guimaraens D, Gonzalez Domingo A (1993)
  Type IV allergy to rubber additives: a 10-year study of 686 cases. J Am
  Acad Dermatol 29:176–180

Hervé-Bazin B, Gradiski D, Duprat P, Marignac B, Foussereau J, Cavelier C,
  Bieber P (1977) Occupational eczema from *N*-isopropyl-*N*′-phenyl-
  paraphenylenediamine (IPPD) and *N*-dimethyl-1,3 butyl-*N*′-phenyl-
  paraphenylenediamine (DMPPD) in tyres. Contact Dermatitis 3:1–15

Von Hintzenstern J, Heese A, Koch HU, Peters KP, Hornstein OP (1991)
  Frequency, spectrum and occupational relevance of type IV allergies to
  rubber chemicals. Contact Dermatitis 24:244–252

245. Ketoprofen

CAS Registry Number
[22071–15–4]

Ketoprofen is an anti-inflammatory drug, used both topically and
systemically. It is above all a photoallergen, responsible for photo-

allergic or photo-worsened contact dermatitis, with sun-induced, progressive, severe, and durable reactions. Recurrent photosensitivity is possible for many years. Photosensitivities are expected to thiophene-phenylketone derivatives such as tiaprofenic acid and suprofen, to ketoprofen esters such as piketoprofen, and to benzophenone derivatives (see above) such as fenofibrate and benzophenone-3. Concomitant photosensitivities – without clinical relevance – have been observed to fenticlor, tetrachlorosalicylanilide, triclosan, tribromsalan, and bithionol.

Suggested Reading

Durbize E, Vigan M, Puzenat E, Girardin P, Adessi B, Desprez P, Humbert P, Laurent R, Aubin F (2003) Spectrum of cross-photosensitization in 18 consecutive patients with contact photoallergy to ketoprofen: associated photoallergies to non-benzophenone-containing molecules. Contact Dermatitis 48:144–149

Le Coz CJ, Bottlaender A, Scrivener JN, Santinelli F, Cribier BJ, Heid E, Grosshans EM (1998) Photocontact dermatitis from ketoprofen and tiaprofenic acid: cross-reactivity study in 12 consecutive patients. Contact Dermatitis 38:245–252

Le Coz CJ, El Aboubi S, Lefèbvre C, Heid E, Grosshans E (2000) Topical ketoprofen induces persistent and recurrent photosensitivity. Contact Dermatitis 42 [Suppl 2]:46

Le Coz CJ, El Aboubi S, Lefèbvre C, Heid E, Grosshans E (2000) Photoallergy from topical ketoprofen: a clinical, allergological and photobiological study. Contact Dermatitis 42 [Suppl 2]:47

246. Labetalol

CAS Registry Number [36894–69–6]

This beta-adrenergic and alpha-1 blocking agent caused contact dermatitis and a contact anaphylactoid reaction during patch testing in a nurse.

Suggested Reading

Bause GS, Kugelman LC (1990) Contact anaphylactoid response to labetalol. Contact Dermatitis 23:51

247. Lactucin

CAS Registry Number [1891–29–8]

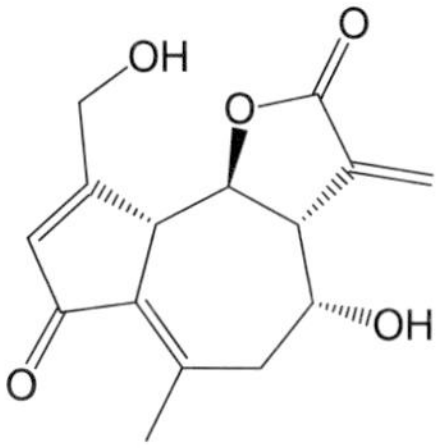

Lactucin, as lactucopicrin, is a sesquiterpene lactone contained in lettuce (*Lactuca sativa* L.).

Suggested Reading

Paulsen E, Andersen KE, Hausen BM (1993) Compositae dermatitis in a Danish dermatology department in one year (I). Results of routine patch testing with the sesquiterpene lactone mix supplemented with aimed patch testing with extracts and sesquiterpene lactones of Compositae plants. Contact Dermatitis 29 : 6–10

248. Lactucopicrin

Intybin

CAS Registry Number [6466–74–6]

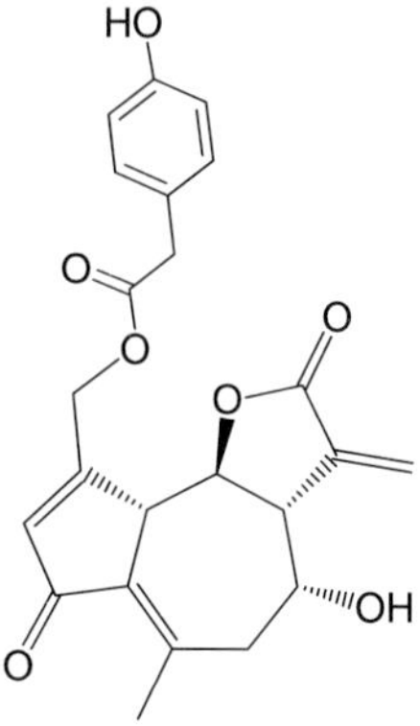

Lactucopicrin, as lactucin, is a sesquiterpene lactone extracted from various *Lactuca* spp. and *Cichorium intybus* L., Asteraceae–Compositae family.

Suggested Reading

Bischoff TA, Kelley CJ, Karchesy Y, Laurantos M, Nguyen-Dinh P, Arefi AG (2004) Antimalarial activity of lactucin and lactucopicrin: sesquiterpene lactones isolated from *Cichorium intybus* L. J Ethnopharmacol 95:455–457

249. Lapachenol

CAS Registry Number [573–13–7]

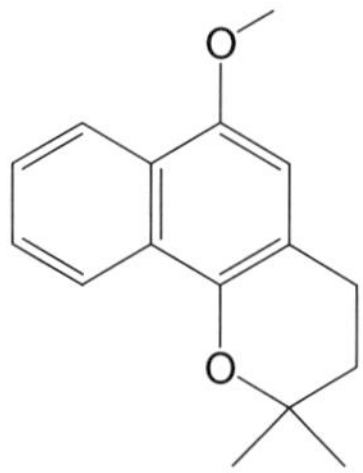

Lapachenol is contained in the heart-wood of Lapacho wood (*Tabebuia avellanedae* Lorentz, Bignoniaceae family). It is a secondary allergen, after lapachol and deoxylapachol, and likely a prohapten transformed in vivo into a quinone hapten.

Suggested Reading

Hausen BM (1981) Wood injurious to human health. A manual. De Gruyter, Berlin

250. Lapachol

**2-Hydroxy-3-(3-Methyl-2-Butenyl)-1,4-Naphthoquinone,
CI 75490,
CI Natural Yellow 16**

CAS Registry Number [84–79–7]

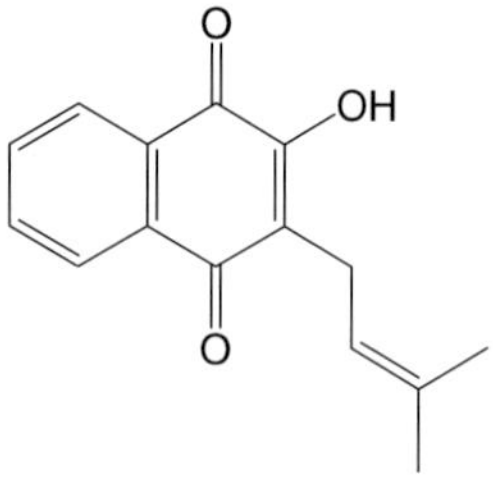

Lapachol, a benzoquinone, is a secondary allergen in teak (*Tectona grandis* L., Verbenaceae family), a wood largely used for various indoor and outdoor applications (doors, windows, etc.) because of its strong durability. It has similar reactivity to deoxylapachol.

Suggested Reading

Estlander T, Jolanki R, Alanko K, Kanerva L (2001) Occupational allergic contact dermatitis caused by wood dusts. Contact Dermatitis 44: 213–217

Lamminpää A, Estlander T, Jolanki R, Kanerva L (1996) Occupational allergic contact dermatitis caused by decorative plants. Contact Dermatitis 34:330–335

251. Lawsone

2-Hydroxy-1,4-Naphthalenedione, Henna

CAS Registry Number [83–72–7]

Henna, prepared by powdering the dried leaves of henna plant (*Lawsonia inermis* L.), is used for coloring and conditioning hair and nails, particularly by Muslims or Hindus. It contains Lawsone, which very rarely induces contact allergy. Most dermatitis caused by "black henna" is due to PPD and derivatives.

Suggested Reading

Le Coz CJ, Lefebvre C, Keller F, Grosshans E (2000) Allergic contact dermatitis caused by skin painting (pseudotattooing) with black henna, a mixture of henna and *p*-phenylenediamine and its derivatives. Arch Dermatol 136:1515–1517

Pasricha JS, Gupta R, Panjwani S (1980) Contact dermatitis to henna (*Lawsonia*). Contact Dermatitis 6:288–290

252. Lidocaine

Lidocaine

CAS Registry Number
[137–58–6]

Lidocaine Hydrochloride Monohydrate

CAS Registry Number [6108–05–0]

Lidocaine is an anesthetic of the amide group, like articaine or bupivacaine. Immediate-type IgE-dependent reactions are rare, and delayed-type contact dermatitis is exceptional. Cross reactivity between the different amide anesthetics is not systematic.

Suggested Reading

Duque S, Fernandez L (2004) Delayed hypersensitivity to amide local anaesthetics. Allergol Immunopathol (Madr) 32 : 233–234

Waton J, Boulanger A, Trechot PH, Schmutz JL, Barbaud A (2004) Contact urticaria from Emla® cream. Contact Dermatitis 51 : 284–287

253. Lilial®

See 73. *p-tert*-Butyl-alpha-Methylhydrocinnamic Aldehyde

254. Limonene

Limonene: D-Limonene + L-Limonene

CAS Registry Number [138–86–3]

D-Limonene: (+)-Limonene, *R*-Limonene, α-Limonene, (*R*)-*p*-Mentha-1,8-Diene, Dipentene, Carvene, Citrene

CAS Registry Number [5989–27–5]

L-Limonene: (–)-Limonene, *S*-Limonene, β-Limonene, (4*S*)-1-Methyl-4-(1-Methylethenyl)-Cyclohexene

CAS Registry Number
[5989–54–8]

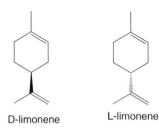

D-limonene   L-limonene

Limonene is a racemic form of D- and L-limonene. D-Limonene is contained in *Citrus* species such as citrus, orange, mandarin, and bergamot. L-Limonene is contained in *Pinus pinea*. The racemic form (D- and L-limonene) is also named dipentene. D-limonene, used as a solvent, may be found in cleansing or in degreasing agents. Its sensitizing potential increases with prolonged air contact, which induces oxidation and leads to oxidation products. The presence of D-limonene has to be mentioned by name in cosmetics of the EU.

Suggested Reading

Karlberg AT, Magnusson K, Nilsson U (1992) Air oxidation of d-limonene (the citrus solvent) creates potent allergens. Contact Dermatitis 26: 332–340

Karlberg AT, Dooms-Goossens A (1997) Contact allergy to oxidized d-limonene among dermatitis patients. Contact Dermatitis 36:201–206

Meding B, Barregard L, Marcus K (1994) Hand eczema in car mechanics. Contact Dermatitis 30:129–134

255. Linalool

3,7-Dimethyl-1,6-octadien-3-ol, Linalyl alcohol,
2,6-Dimethyl-2,7-octadien-6-ol

CAS Registry Number [78–70–6]

Linalool is a terpene chief constituent of linaloe oil, also found in oils of Ceylon cinnamon, sassafras, orange flower, bergamot, *Artemisia balchanorum*, ylang-ylang. This frequently used scented substance is a sensitizer by the way of primary or secondary oxidation products. As a fragrance allergen, linalool has to be mentioned by name in cosmetics within the EU.

Suggested Reading

Kanerva L, Estlander T, Jolanki R (1995) Occupational allergic contact dermatitis caused by ylang-ylang oil. Contact Dermatitis 33:198–199

Skold M, Borje A, Harambasic E, Karlberg AT (2004) Contact allergens formed on air exposure of linalool. Identification and quantification of primary and secondary oxidation products and the effect on skin sensitization. Chem Res Toxicol 17:1697–1705

256. Lincomycin (Hydrochloride Monohydrate)

Lincomycin

CAS Registry Number
[154–21–2]

Lincomycin Hydrochloride Monohydrate

CAS Registry Number
[7179–49–9]

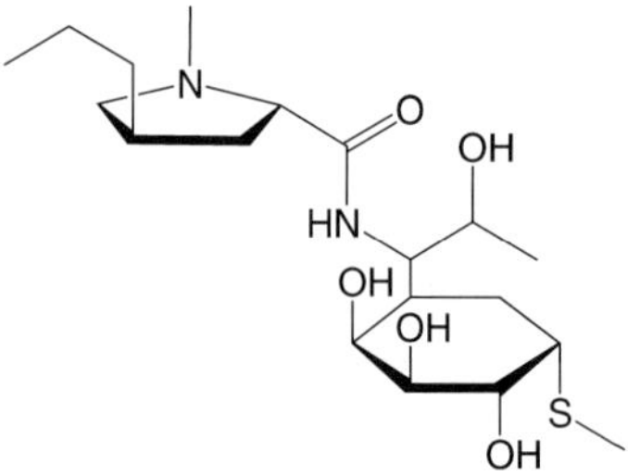

Lincomycin is an antibiotic of the lincosanide group, active against Gram-positive bacteria. Occupational exposure occurs in poultry and pig breeders.

Suggested Reading

Vilaplana J, Romaguera C, Grimalt F (1991) Contact dermatitis from lincomycin and spectinomycin in chicken vaccinators. Contact Dermatitis 24:225–226

257. Lindane

γ-1,2,3,4,5,6-Hexachlorocyclohexane

CAS Registry Number [58–89–9]

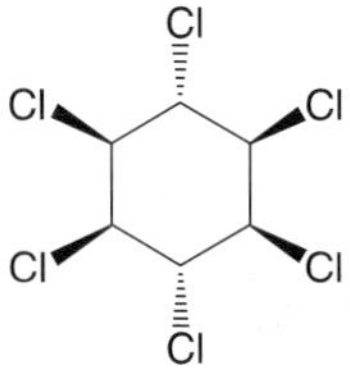

Lindane is a pesticide used for its anti-insect properties in agriculture, wood protection, in anti-insect paints, and veterinary and human medicine against many insects such as spiders, mosquitoes, ticks, scabies, lice, and demodicidosis. Its use is controlled, particularly because of neurological toxicity.

Suggested Reading

Anonymous (1992) Fiche toxicologique n°81. Cahiers documentaires de l'INRS

Sharma VK, Kaur S (1990) Contact sensitization by pesticides in farmers. Contact Dermatitis 23:77–80

258. Lyral®

See 236. Hydroxymethylpentacyclohexenecarboxaldehyde

259. Malathion

Carbetox, Carbofos, Chemathion, Cimexan, Dorthion, Extermathion, Fosfotion

CAS Registry Number [121–75–5]

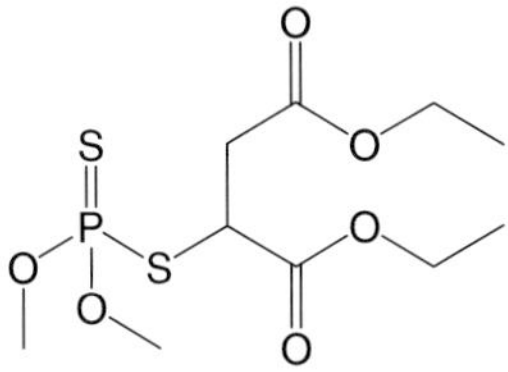

This organophosphorus pesticide is used as an insecticide and an acaricide, particularly against head lice. Sensitization was reported in farmers.

Suggested Reading

O'Malley M, Rodriguez P, Maibach HI (1995) Pesticide patch testing: California nursery workers and controls. Contact Dermatitis 32 : 61–62

Sharma VK, Kaur S (1990) Contact sensitization by pesticides in farmers. Contact Dermatitis 23 : 77–80

260. Mancozeb

Zinc Manganese Ethylenebisdithiocarbamate

CAS Registry Number [8018–01–7]

Mancozeb is a fungicide of the ethylene-bis-dithiocarbamate group. It is present in Rondo-M® with pyrifenox. Occupational exposure occurs mainly in agricultural workers, in vineyard workers or in florists.

Suggested Reading

Crippa M, Misquith L, Lonati A, Pasolini G (1990) Dyshidrotic eczema and sensitization to dithiocarbamates in a florist. Contact Dermatitis 23 : 203–204

Iliev D, Elsner P (1997) Allergic contact from the fungicide Rondo-M® and the insecticide Alfacron®. Contact Dermatitis 36 : 51

Jung HD, Honemann W, Kloth C, Lubbe D, Pambor M, Quednow C, Ratz KH, Rothe A, Tarnick M (1989) Kontaktekzem durch Pestizide in der Deutschen Demokratischen Republik. Dermatol Monatsschr 175 : 203–214

Koch P (1996) Occupational allergic contact dermatitis and airborne contact dermatitis from 5 fungicides in a vineyard worker. Cross-reactions between fungicides of the dithiocarbamate group? Contact Dermatitis 34 : 324–329

261. Maneb

Ethylenebisdithiocarbamate Manganese

CAS Registry Number [12427–38–2]

Maneb is a pesticide with fungicide properties, belonging to the dithiocarbamate group. Sensitization occurs mainly in farmers and agricultural workers.

Suggested Reading

Crippa M, Misquith L, Lonati A, Pasolini G (1990) Dyshidrotic eczema and sensitization to dithiocarbamates in a florist. Contact Dermatitis 23: 203–204

Jung HD, Honemann W, Kloth C, Lubbe D, Pambor M, Quednow C, Ratz KH, Rothe A, Tarnick M (1989) Kontaktekzem durch Pestizide in der Deutschen Demokratischen Republik. Dermatol Monatsschr 175: 203–214

Koch P (1996) Occupational allergic contact dermatitis and airborne contact dermatitis from 5 fungicides in a vineyard worker. Cross-reactions between fungicides of the dithiocarbamate group? Contact Dermatitis 34:324–329

O'Malley M, Rodriguez P, Maibach HI (1995) Pesticide patch testing: California nursery workers and controls. Contact Dermatitis 32:61–62

Peluso AM, Tardio M, Adamo F, Venturo N (1991) Multiple sensitization due to bis-dithiocarbamate and thiophthalimide pesticides. Contact Dermatitis 25:327

Piraccini BM, Cameli N, Peluso AM, Tardio M (1991) A case of allergic contact dermatitis due to the pesticide maneb. Contact Dermatitis 24: 381–382

Sharma VK, Kaur S (1990) Contact sensitization by pesticides in farmers. Contact Dermatitis 23:77–80

262. Melamine and Melamine-Formaldehyde Resins

Melamine: 2,4,6-Triaminotriazine

CAS Registry Number
[108–78–1]

Melamine-formaldehyde resin (MFR) result from condensation of melamine and formaldehyde. It is an active ingredient of strong (reinforced) plasters, such as industrial or some dental plasters used for moulding. It is also used as a textile finish resin. MFR acts as an allergen generally because of formaldehyde releasing).

Suggested Reading

Aalto-Korte K, Jolanki R, Estlander T (2003) Formaldehyde-negative allergic contact dermatitis from melamine-formaldehyde resin. Contact Dermatitis 49 : 194–196

Garcia Bracamonte B, Ortiz de Frutos FJ, Iglesias Diez L (1995) Occupational allergic contact dermatitis due to formaldehyde and textile finish resins. Contact Dermatitis 33 : 139–140

Lewis FM, Cork MJ, McDonagh AJG, Gawkrodger DJG (1993) Allergic contact dermatitis from resin-reinforced plaster. Contact Dermatitis 28 : 40–41

Rustemeyer T, Frosch PJ (1996) Occupational skin diseases in dental laboratory technicians. (I). Clinical picture and causative factors. Contact Dermatitis 34 : 125–133

263. Mercaptobenzothiazole

2-Mercaptobenzothiazole, MBT

CAS Registry Number
[149–30–4]

MBT is a rubber chemical, accelerant of vulcanization, and contained in "mercapto-mix." The most frequent occupational categories are the metal industry, homemakers, health services and laboratories, the building industry, and shoemakers. It is also used as a corrosion inhibitor in cutting fluids or in releasing fluids in the pottery industry.

Suggested Reading

Condé-Salazar L, Del-Rio E, Guimaraens D, Gonzalez Domingo A (1993) Type IV allergy to rubber additives: a 10-year study of 686 cases. J Am Acad Dermatol 29:176–180

Mancuso G, Reggiani M, Berdondini RM (1996) Occupational dermatitis in shoemakers. Contact Dermatitis 34:17–22

Von Hintzenstern J, Heese A, Koch HU, Peters KP, Hornstein OP (1991) Frequency, spectrum and occupational relevance of type IV allergies to rubber chemicals. Contact Dermatitis 24:244–252

Wilkinson SM, Cartwright PH, English JSC (1990) Allergic contact dermatitis from mercaptobenzothiazole in a releasing fluid. Contact Dermatitis 23:370

264. Mercaptobenzothiazole Salts

Mercaptobenzothiazole, Sodium Salt

CAS Registry Numbers [2492-26-4]

Mercaptobenzothiazole, Zinc Salt

CAS Registry Numbers [155-04-4]

Such mercaptobenzothiazole hydrosoluble salts are used as antioxidants and biocides in cutting fluids and greases, paints or glues.

Suggested Reading

Le Coz CJ (2004) Fiche d'éviction en cas d'hypersensibilité au mercapto-benzothiazole et au mercapto mix. Ann Dermatol Venereol 131: 1012–1014

265. MESNA

Sodium 2-Mercaptoethane Sulfonate

CAS Registry Number [19767–45–4]

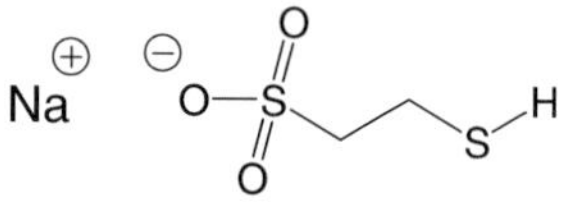

Mesna is used as a mucolytic agent, and as an antidote to chloro-acetyl-aldehyde and acrolein (a bladder toxic metabolite of ifosfamide or cyclophosphamide). It has been reported as a cause of occupational allergic (hand and airborne) dermatitis in nurses.

Suggested Reading

Benyoussef K, Bottlaender A, Pfister HR, Caussade P, Heid E, Grosshans E (1996) Allergic contact dermatitis from mesna. Contact Dermatitis 34: 228–229

Kiec-Swierczynska M, Krecisz B (2003) Occupational airborne allergic contact dermatitis from mesna. Contact Dermatitis 48:171

266. Metacresol

3-Cresol, 3-Methylphenol, *m*-Cresol

CAS Registry Number [108–39–4]

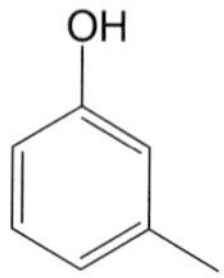

Metacresol is contained as a preservative in almost all human insulin. It has been reported as a cause of allergic reaction due to injected insulin.

Suggested Reading

Clerx V, van den Keybus C, Kochuyt A, Goossens A (2003) Drug intolerance reaction to insulin therapy caused by metacresol. Contact Dermatitis 48:162–163

267. Metanil Yellow

Acid Yellow 36, CI 13065

CAS Registry Number [587–98–4]

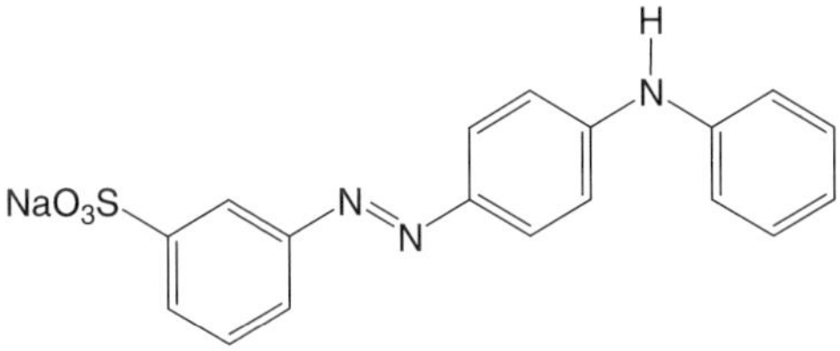

Metanil yellow is a yellow monoazoic dye. This coloring agent used in leather and wood stains, and was also employed as a food dye in India.

Suggested Reading

Hausen BM (1994) A case of allergic contact dermatitis due to metanil yellow. Contact Dermatitis 31 : 117–118

268. Methenamine

Hexamethylenetetramine

CAS Registry Number [100–97–0]

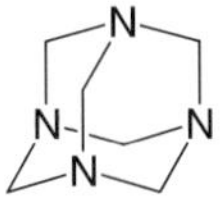

Hexamethylenetetramine is used in the foundry, tire and rubber, and phenol formaldehyde resins industries and in other applications such as a hardener in epoxy resins Bisphenol A type and as an anticorrosive agent. It is an ammonia and formaldehyde releaser sometimes used in topical medicaments and cosmetics.

Suggested Reading

Gonzalez-Perez R, Gonzalez-Hermosa R, Aseginolaza B, Luis Diaz-Ramon J, Soloeta R (2003) Allergic contact dermatitis from methenamine in an antiperspirant spray. Contact Dermatitis 49 : 266

Holness DL, Nethercott JR (1993) The performance of specialized collections of bisphenol A epoxy resin system components in the evaluation of workers in an occupational health clinic population. Contact Dermatitis 28 : 216–219

269. Methidathion

Somonil, Supracid, Suprathion, Ultracid

CAS Registry Number [950–37–8]

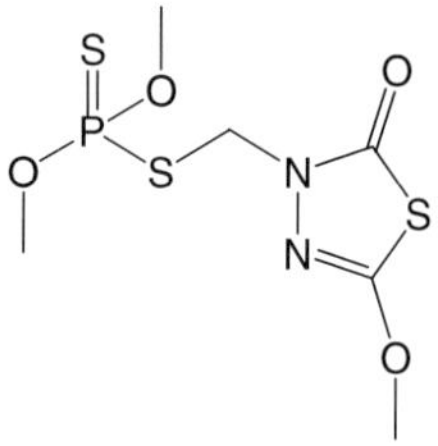

Methidation is an organophosphorus compound used as an insecticide. Cross-sensitivity was described to Dichlorvos.

Suggested Reading

Ueda A, Aoyama K, Manda F, Ueda T, Kawahara Y (1994) Delayed-type allergenicity of triforine (Saprol®). Contact Dermatitis 31:140–145

270. Methiocarb

3,5-Dimethyl-4-(Methylthio)Phenol Methylcarbamate, Mesurol

CAS Registry Number [2032–65–7]

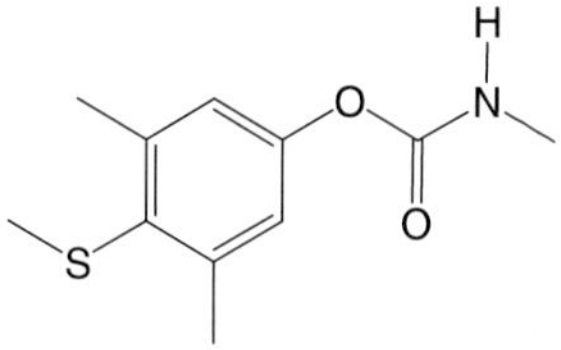

Methiocarb is an insecticide or molluscicide with a cholinesterase inhibiting effect. A case of contact dermatitis was reported in a carnation grower.

Suggested Reading

Willems PWJM, Geursen-Reitsma AM, van Joost T (1997) Allergic contact dermatitis due to methiocarb (Mesurol). Contact Dermatitis 36:270

271. Methomyl

S-Methyl-N-(Methylcarbamoyloxy)-Thioacetimidate, Lannate

CAS Registry Number [16752–77–5]

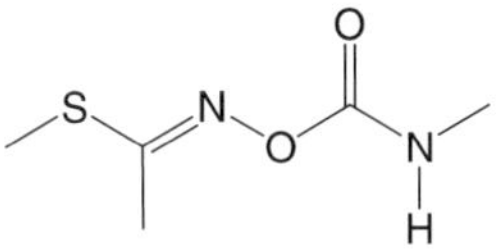

Methomyl is a pesticide agent, a carbamate insecticide with anticholinesterase activity. This mixture of two stereoisomers is used as a foliar spray to control field crops, stables and poultry houses, and in glasshouses on ornamentals and vegetables, or in flypapers. Cases were reported in chrysanthemum growers and in two women working in a plant nursery.

Suggested Reading

Bruynzeel DP (1991) Contact sensitivity to Lannate®. Contact Dermatitis 25:60–61

272. (R)-4-Methoxy Dalbergione

CAS Registry Number [4640–26–0] [28396–75–0]

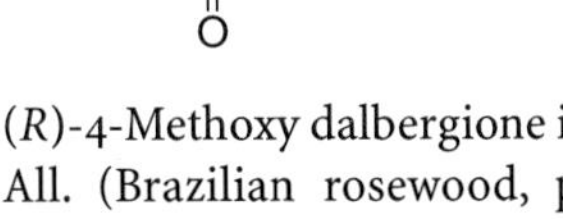

(R)-4-Methoxy dalbergione is the main allergen of *Dalbergia nigra* All. (Brazilian rosewood, palissander) and *Dalbergia latifolia* Roxb. (East Indian rosewood). Occupational sensitization occurs in timber workers.

Suggested Reading

Gallo R, Guarrera M, Hausen BM (1996) Airborne contact dermatitis from East Indian rosewood (*Dalbergia latifolia* Roxb.). Contact Dermatitis 35:60–61

Hausen BM (2000) Woods. In: Kanerva L, Elsner P, Wahlberg JE, Maibach
HI (eds) Handbook of occupational dermatology. Springer, Berlin
Heidelberg New York, pp 771–780

273. Methoxy PEG-17/Dodecyl Glycol Copolymer

CAS Registry Number
[88507–00–0]

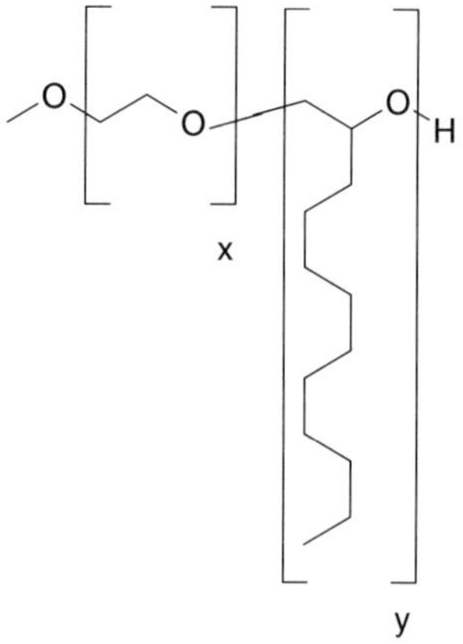

Methoxy PEG-17/dodecyl glycol copolymer is one of the numerous
copolymers recorded in the International Nomenclature of Cosmetics Ingredients (INCI) inventory system. It belongs to the chemical class of alkoxylated alcohols. It is utilized as an emulsion
stabilizer, a skin-conditioning and a viscosity-increasing agent in
cosmetics.

Suggested Reading
Le Coz CJ, Heid E (2001) Allergic contact dermatitis from methoxy PEG-
17/dodecyl glycol copolymer (Elfacos® OW 100). Contact Dermatitis
44:308–309

274. Methoxy-Psoralens

5-Methoxypsoralen, Bergapten(e)

CAS Registry Number [484–20–8]

8-Methoxypsoralen, Methoxsalen, Meladinin, Xanthotoxin

CAS Registry Number [298–81–7]

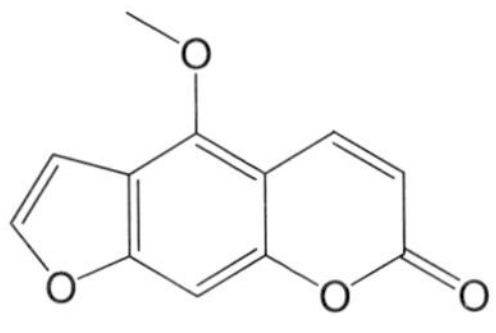

5-MOP 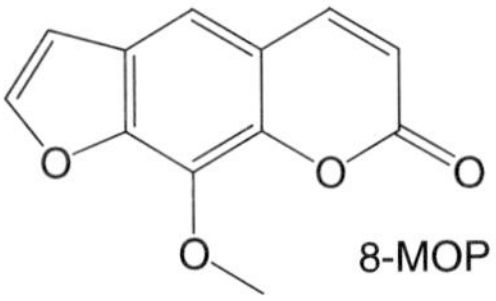   8-MOP

These fur(an)ocoumarins are phototoxic compounds that cause phototoxic dermatitis. Many plants of the Apiaceae–Umbelliferae and most of the Rutaceae family contain 5-methoxypsoralen and 8-methoxypsoralen. Their spectra is in the UVA range (300–360 nm). They are used in combination with UVA to treat various skin disorders such as psoriasis.

Suggested Reading

Ena P, Camarda I (1990) Phytophotodermatitis from *Ruta corsica*. Contact Dermatitis 22:63

Ena P, Cerri R, Dessi G, Manconi PM, Atzei AD (1991) Phototoxicity due to *Cachrys libanotis*. Contact Dermatitis 24:1–5

275. Methyl 2,3 Epoxy-3-(4-Methoxyphenyl)Propionate

3-(-Methoxyphenyl)Glycidic Acid Methylester, Methyl 3-(p-Methoxyphenyl)Oxirane-2-Carboxylate

CAS Registry Number [42245–42–1]

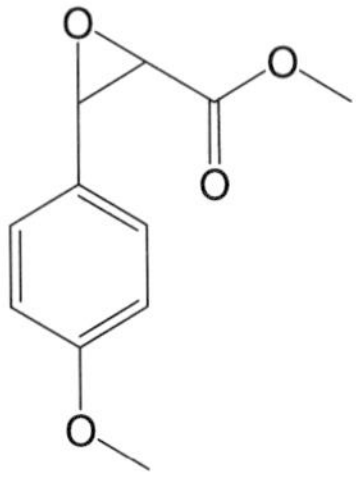

Methyl 2,3 epoxy-3-(4-methoxyphenyl)propionate is an intermediate product in the synthesis of diltiazem hydrochloride. Contact dermatitis was observed in several laboratory technicians.

Suggested Reading
Rudzki E, Rebandel P (1990) Dermatitis from methyl 2,3 epoxy-3-(4-methoxyphenyl)propionate. Contact Dermatitis 23 : 382

276. Methyl Gallate

CAS Registry Number [99–24–1]

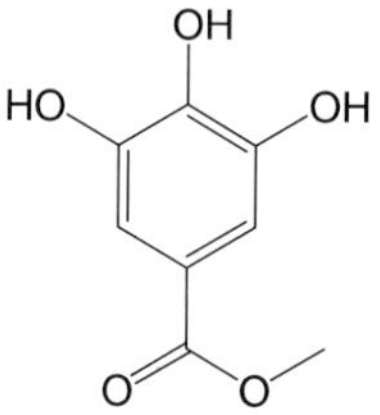

This ester of gallic acid is used as an antioxidant agent. A case was reported by using a reprography paper.

Suggested Reading
Degos R, Lépine J, Akhoundzadeh H (1968) Sensibilisation cutanée due à la manipulation de papier reprographie. Bull Soc Fr Dermatol 75 : 595–596

277. Methyl Heptine Carbonate

Methyl oct-2-ynoate, Folione

CAS Registry Number [111–12–6]

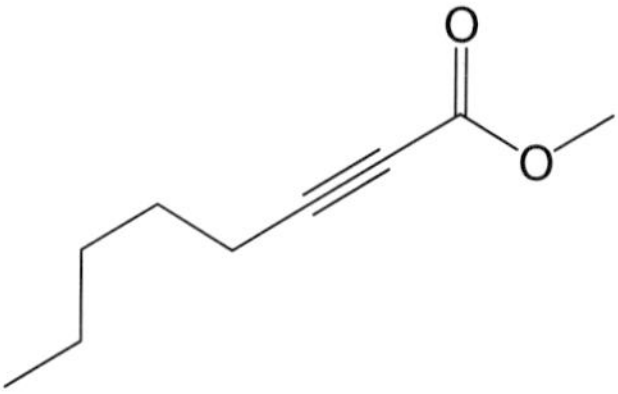

This perfumed molecule belongs to the list of 26 allergens that have to be indicated by name on the ingredients list of cosmetics in the EU.

Suggested Reading
English JS, Rycroft RJ (1988) Allergic contact dermatitis from methyl heptine and methyl octine carbonates. Contact Dermatitis 18 : 174–175

278. Methyl Octine Carbonate

Methyl non-2-ynoate

CAS Registry Number
[111–80–8]

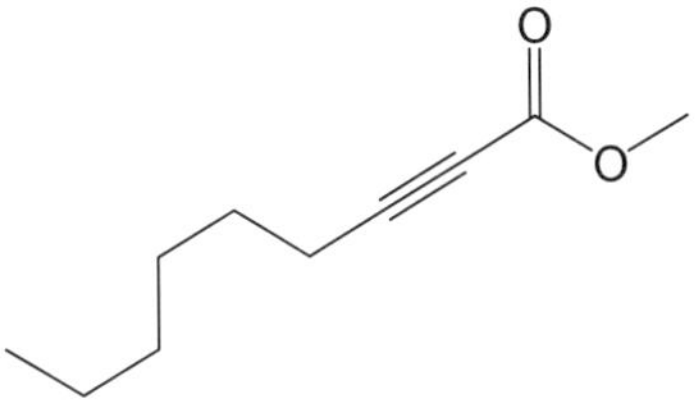

This perfumed molecule is related to methyl heptine carbonate. Cross-reactivity is frequent.

Suggested Reading

English JS, Rycroft RJ (1988) Allergic contact dermatitis from methyl heptine and methyl octine carbonates. Contact Dermatitis 18:174–175

279. Methyl Salicylate

CAS Registry Number [119–36–8]

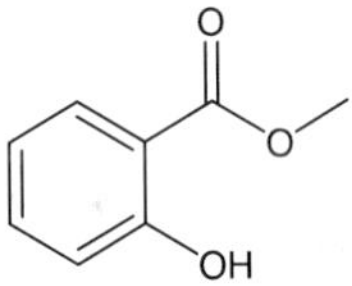

This anti-inflammatory agent is found in a wide number of ointments and can induce allergic contact dermatitis.

Suggested Reading

Hindson C (1977) Contact eczema from methyl salicylate reproduced by oral aspirin (acetyl salicylic acid). Contact Dermatitis 3:348–349

Oiso N, Fulai K, Ishii M (2004) Allergic contact dermatitis due to methyl salicylate in a compress. Contact Dermatitis 51:34–35

280. Methyl-Terpyridine

2,2′: 6′,2″-(4′-Methyl)-*ter*-Pyridine),
4′-Methyl (2,2′,2″-Terpyridine)

CAS Registry Number for 2,2′,2″-Terpyridine [1148–79–4]

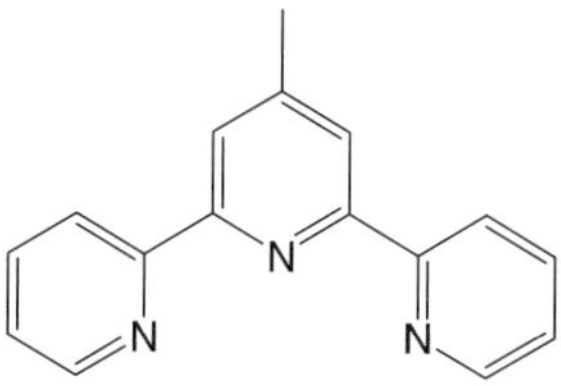

This molecule is a terpyridine with a 4′-methyl substitution. A case of occupational dermatitis was reported in a chemical technician with no cross-reactivity to pyridine derivatives.

Suggested Reading
Le Coz CJ, Caussade P, Bottlaender A (1998) Occupational contact dermatitis from methyl-*ter*-pyridine in a chemistry laboratory technician. Contact Dermatitis 38 : 214–215

281. 2-Methyl-4,5-Trimethylene-4-Isothiazolin-3-one

CAS Registry Number [82633–79–2]

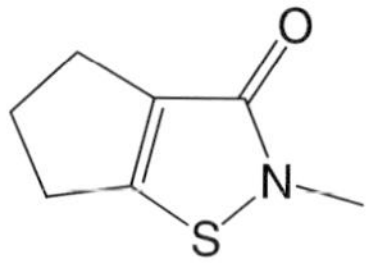

This biocide induced contact dermatitis in a laboratory technician, also sensitive to the other isothiazolinone BIT.

Suggested Reading
Burden AD, O'Driscoll JB, Page FC, Beck MH (1994) Contact hypersensitivity to a new isothiazolinone. Contact Dermatitis 30 : 179–180

282. Methylchloroisothiazolinone

Chloromethylisothiazolinone, 5-Chloro-2-Methyl-4-Isothiazolin-3-one, MCI

CAS Registry Number [26172–55–4]

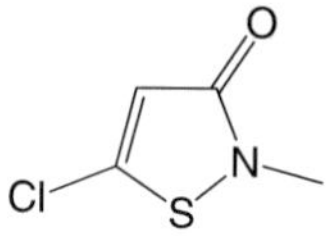

MCI is mainly associated with methylisothiazolinone for its bactericidal and fongistatic properties. It is found in Kathon® CG or derivatives. MCI is found in water-based products such as cosmetics, paints, and glues. Pure MCI is highly irritant and may cause active sensitization.

Suggested Reading

Nielsen H (1994) Occupational exposure to isothiazolinones. A study based on a product register. Contact Dermatitis 31:18–21

Schubert H (1997) Airborne contact dermatitis due to methylchloro- and methylisothiazolinone (MCI/MI). Contact Dermatitis 36:274

Tay P, Ng SK (1994) Delayed skin burns from MCI/MI biocide used in water treatment. Contact Dermatitis 30:54–55

283. Methylchloroisothiazolinone + Methylsiothiazolinone (MCI/MI)

CAS Registry Numbers [55965–84–9], [96118–96–6]

Kathon® CG (CG = Cosmetic Grade) is a 3:1 mixture of CMI and MI, at a 1.5% concentration. It is used for cosmetics and toiletries, metalworking fluids or paints, in which it can be added only periodically or in color film developers. Kathon® 886 MW (MW = metalworking fluids) is a mixture CMI/MI mixture at a 13.9% concentration, mainly contained in metalworking fluids. Kathon® FP 1.5 contains MCI/MI at 1.5% concentration in propylene glycol. Kathon® LX (LX = LateX) contains MCI/MI at a tenfold concentration of Kathon® CG. Kathon® WT (WT = water treatment) is a MCI/MI mixture used in the paper industry. Parmetol® K40, Parmethol® DF 12 and Parmetol® DF 35, Parmetol® A 23, Parmetol® K50, and Parmetol® DF 18 are other brand names of MCI/MI.

Suggested Reading

Björkner B, Bruze M, Dahlquist I, Fregert S, Gruvberger B, Persson K (1986) Contact allergy to the preservative Kathon® CG. Contact Dermatitis 14:85–90

Fernandez de Corres L, Navarro JA, Gastaminza G, del Pozo MD (1995) An
    unusual case of sensitization to methylchloro- and methyl-isothiazol-
    inone (MCI/MI). Contact Dermatitis 33:215
Pazzaglia M, Vincenzi C, Gasparri F, Tosti A (1996) Occupational hyper-
    sensitivity to isothiazolinone derivatives in a radiology technician.
    Contact Dermatitis 34:143–144
Scheman AJ, Katta R (1997) Photographic allergens: an update. Contact
    Dermatitis 37:130

284. Methyldibromoglutaronitrile

1,2-Dibromo 2,4-Dicyanobutane

CAS Registry Number [35691–65–7]

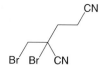

Methyldibromoglutaronitrile is a biocide widely used as a preservative agent in cosmetics, toiletries, and metalworking fluids. It is
a potent allergen.

Suggested Reading

Aalto-Korte K, Jolanki R, Estlander T, Alanko K, Kanerva L (1996) Occupa-
    tional allergic contact dermatitis caused by Euxyl K 400. Contact
    Dermatitis 35:193–194
Kynemund Pedersen L, Agner T, Held E, Johansen JD (2004) Methyldi-
    bromoglutaronitrile in leave-on products elicits contact allergy at low
    concentration. Br J Dermatol 151:817–822
Le Coz CJ (2005) Hypersensibilité au méthyldibromoglutaronitrile
    (Dibromodicyanobutane). Ann Dermatol Venereol 132:496–497

285. Methylhexahydrophthalic Anhydride

1,3-Isobenzofurandione, Hexahydromethyl

**CAS Registry Numbers [19438–60–9] [39363–62–7],
[86403–41–0], [95032–44–3]**

Methylhexahydrophthalic anhydride is an epoxy hardener, irritant to skin and mucous membranes. It is included in non-diglycidyl-ether-of-bisphenol-A epoxy resins. It can induce both allergic contact dermatitis and immunologic contact urticaria. It is structurally close to methyltetrahydrophthalic anhydride, which can also cause sensitization.

Suggested Reading

Kanerva L, Jolanki R, Estlander T (1997) Allergic contact dermatitis from non-diglycidyl-ether-of-bisphenol-A epoxy resins. Contact Dermatitis 36:34–38

Tarvainen K, Jolanki R, Estlander T, Tupasela O, Pfäffli P, Kanerva L (1995) Immunologic contact urticaria due to airborne methylhexahydrophthalic and methyltetrahydrophthalic anhydrides. Contact Dermatitis 32:204–209

286. Methylisothiazolinone

2-Methyl-4-Isothiazolin-3-one, MI

CAS Registry Number [2682–20–4]

MI is generally associated with MCI, in Kathon® CG, MCI/MI, and Euxyl® K 100. This preservative is currently used in water-based products such as cosmetics, paints, and glues. Skin contact with concentrated solution can cause severe irritant dermatitis.

Suggested Reading

Schubert H (1997) Airborne contact dermatitis due to methylchloro- and methylisothiazolinone (MCI/MI). Contact Dermatitis 36:274

Tay P, Ng SK (1994) Delayed skin burns from MCI/MI biocide used in water treatment. Contact Dermatitis 30:54–55

287. Methylol Phenols

2-Methylol Phenol: 2-Hydroxymethyl-Phenol

CAS Registry Number [90–01–7]

3-Methylol Phenol: 3-Hydroxymethyl-Phenol, 3-Hydroxybenzyl Alcohol

CAS Registry Number [620–24–6]

4-Methylol Phenol: 4-Hydroxymethyl-Phenol

CAS Registry Number [623–05–2]

OH OH   OH   OH

2-MP   OH   4-MP
                   3-MP   OH

Methylol phenols are sensitizers contained in resins based on phenol and formaldehyde of the resol type. Cross-reactivity is possible with other phenol derivative molecules.

Suggested Reading

Bruze M, Zimerson E (1997) Cross-reaction patterns in patients with contact allergy to simple methylol phenols. Contact Dermatitis 37:82–86

Bruze M, Fregert S, Zimerson E (1985) Contact allergy to phenol-formaldehyde resins. Contact Dermatitis 12:81–86

288. 1-Methylpyrrolidone

N-Methyl-2-Pyrrolidone, 1-Methyl-2-Pyrrolidone

CAS Registry Number [872–50–4].

1-Methylpyrrolidone is an aprotic solvent with a wide range of applications: petrochemical processing, surface coating, dyes and pigments, industrial and domestic cleaning compounds, and agricultural and pharmaceutical formulations. It is mainly an irritant, but it can cause severe contact dermatitis due to prolonged contact.

Suggested Reading

Jungbauer FH, Coenraads PJ, Kardaun SH (2001) Toxic hygroscopic contact reaction to N-methyl-2-pyrrolidone. Contact Dermatitis 45:303–304

Leira H, Tiltnes A, Svendsen K, Vetlesen L (1992) Irritant cutaneous reactions to N-methyl-2-pyrrolidone (NMP). Contact Dermatitis 27:148–150

289. Metol (Sulfate)

4(Methylamino)Phenol

CAS Registry Number [150–75–4]

4(Methylamino)Phenol Sulfate

CAS Registry Numbers [1936–57–8] (unspecified sulfate), [51–72–9] (sulfate[1:1]), [55–55–0] (sulfate[2:1])

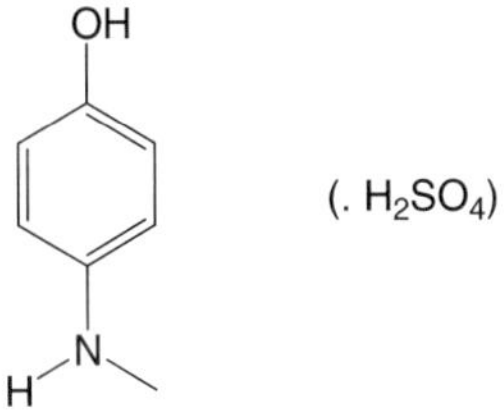

(. H_2SO_4)

Metol is contained in black and white film developers and caused contact dermatitis in photographers.

Suggested Reading

Liden C, Brehmer-Andersson E (1988) Occupational dermatoses from colour developing agents. Clinical and histopathological observations. Acta Derm Venereol (Stockh) 68:514–522

Scheman AJ, Katta R (1997) Photographic allergens: an update. Contact Dermatitis 37:130

290. Mevinphos

CAS Registry Number [7786–34–7]

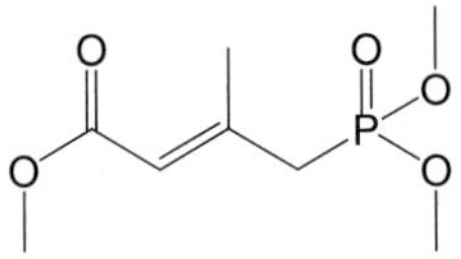

Sensitization to mevinphos (also named Duraphos, Phosdrin, and Phosfene), an organophosphate cholinesterase inhibitor that is used as an insecticide, was rarely reported.

Suggested Reading

Jung HD, Ramsauer E (1987) Akute Pesticid-Intoxication kombiniert mit epicutaner Sensibilisierung durch den organischen Phosphorsäure-ester Mevinphos (PD5). Aktuel Dermatol 13:82–83

291. Mezlocilin

CAS Registry Number [51481–65–3]

Mezlocillin Sodium Salt Monohydrate

CAS Registry Number [59798–30–0]

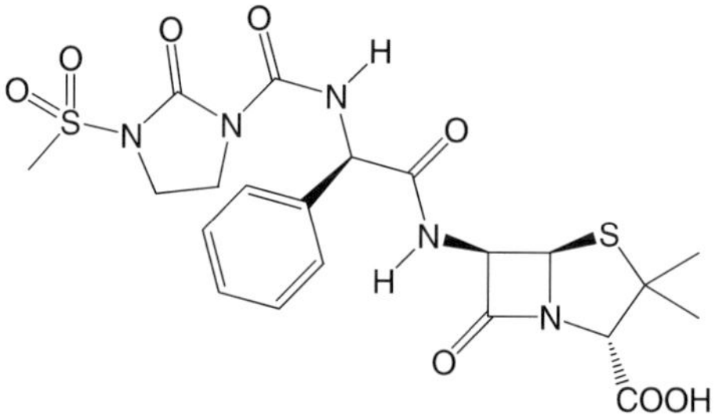

Mezlocillin is an acylaminopenicillin, which caused both immediate and delayed hypersensitivity in a nurse.

Suggested Reading

Keller K, Schwanitz HJ (1992) Combined immediate and delayed hypersensitivity to mezlocillin. Contact Dermatitis 27:348–349

292. Monoethanolamine

Ethanolamine, 2-Aminoethanol

CAS Registry Number [141–43–5]

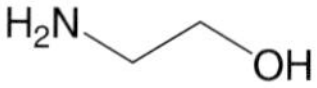

Monoethanolamine is contained in many products, such as metalworking fluids. It is mainly an irritant. Traces may exist in other ethanolamine fluids.

Suggested Reading

Bhushan M, Craven NM, Beck MH (1998) Contact allergy to 2-aminoethanol (monoethanolamine) in a soluble oil. Contact Dermatitis 39: 321

Blum A, Lischka G (1997) Allergic contact dermatitis from mono-, di- and triethanolamine. Contact Dermatitis 36:166

293. Morphine (Morphine Hydrochloride, Morphine Tartrate)

CAS Registry Number [57–27–2] (CAS Registry Number [52–26–6], CAS Registry Number [302–31–8])

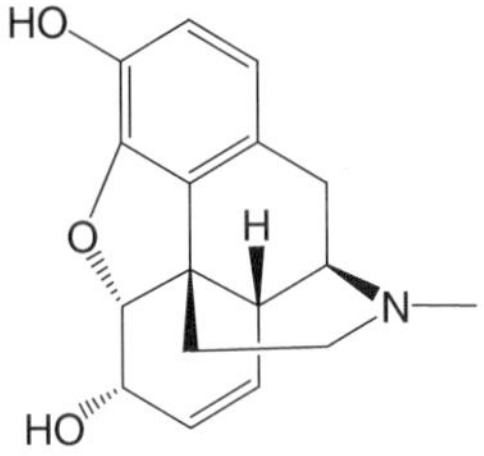

Morphine bitartrate caused contact dermatitis in a worker at a plant producing opium alkaloids. Morphine hydrochloride and morphine bitartrate showed patch-test-positive reactions in another patient with contact dermatitis working in the production of concentrated poppy straw. We observed a concomitant reaction between a morphine base and a codeine base in a patient with drug skin eruption due to codeine.

Suggested Reading

Condé-Salazar L, Guimaraens D, Gonzalez M, Fuente C (1991) Occupational allergic contact dermatitis from opium alkaloids. Contact Dermatitis 25 : 202–203

294. 4-Morpholinyl-2-Benzothiazyle Disulfide

2-(Morpholinodithio)Benzothiazole, Benzothiazole, 2-(4-morpholinyldithio)

CAS Registry Number [95–32–9]

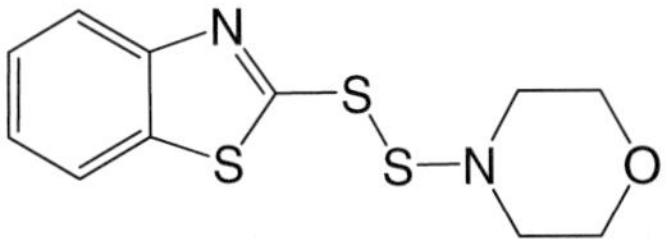

This chemical is a mercaptobenzothiazole-sulfenamide compound, used as moderate accelerator in rubber vulcanization.

Suggested Reading

Le Coz CJ (2004) Fiche d'éviction en cas d'hypersensibilité au mercapto-
    benzothiazole et au mercapto mix. Ann Dermatol Venereol 131:
    1012–1014

295. Morpholinyl Mercaptobenzothiazole

2-(4-Morpholinylthiobenzothiazole),
2-Morpholin Benzothiazyl Sulfenamide, Benzothiazole,
2-(4-Morpholinylthio)

CAS Registry Number [102–77–2]

This rubber vulcanization accelerator belongs to the mercaptobenzothiazole-sulfenamide group. It is used as a chemical in the
rubber industry, especially in the production of synthetic rubber
articles. It is contained in "mercapto mix." As a corrosion inhibitor,
it can be found in cutting fluids or in releasing fluids in the pottery
industry. It induces mainly delayed-type hypersensitivity, but a
case of immediate-type hypersensitivity was reported in a dental
assistant.

Suggested Reading

Brehler R (1996) Contact urticaria caused by latex-free nitrile gloves. Con-
    tact Dermatitis 34:296
Condé-Salazar L, Del-Rio E, Guimaraens D, Gonzalez Domingo A (1993)
    Type IV allergy to rubber additives: a 10-year study of 686 cases. J Am
    Acad Dermatol 29:176–180
Le Coz CJ (2004) Fiche d'éviction en cas d'hypersensibilité au mercapto-
    benzothiazole et au mercapto mix. Ann Dermatol Venereol 131: 131:
    846–848

296. Naled

CAS Registry Number [300–76–5]

Naled is an organophosphate cholinesterase inhibitor that is used as an insecticide and as an acaricide. Sensitization seems to be very rare.

Suggested Reading

Edmundson WF, Davies JE (1967) Occupational dermatitis from naled. Arch Environ Health 15:89–91

Mick DL, Gartin TD, Long KR (1970) A case report: occupational exposure to the insecticide naled. J Iowa Med Soc 60:395–396

297. 1-Naphthol

Alpha-Naphthol, CI 76605, CI Oxidation Base 33

CAS Registry Number [90–15–3]

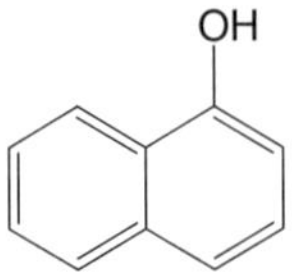

Alpha-naphthol can be used in dye manufacture and is classified as a hair dye. Combined with epichlorhydrin and NaOH to form alpha-naphthyl glycidyl ether, it caused sensitization in one of three workers in a chemical plant.

Suggested Reading

De Groot AC (1994) Occupational contact allergy to alpha-naphthyl glycidyl ether. Contact Dermatitis 30:253–254

298. Naphthol AS

CI 37505, CI Azoic Coupling Component 2

CAS Registry Number [92–77–3]

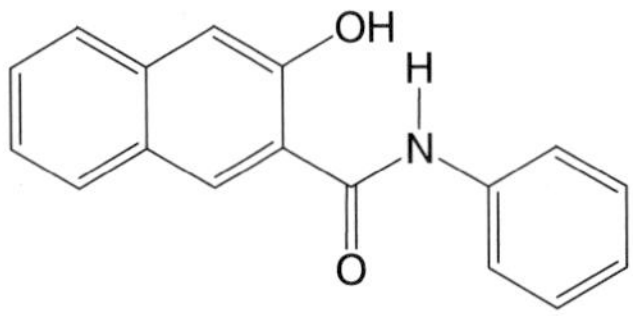

Naphthol AS is a coupling agent in cotton dyeing, inducing occupational dermatitis or contact allergy in consumers in contact with cotton-dyed clothing. It has been indirectly reported as a cause of occupational allergy due to its coupling with Diazo Component 51, or as a cross-sensitizer or sensitizer associated with Pigment Red 23 in red parts of tattoos. Pigmented contact dermatitis is usual in patients with a high phototype.

Suggested Reading

Le Coz CJ, Lepoittevin JP (2001) Clothing dermatitis from Naphthol AS. Contact Dermatitis 44:366–367

Roed-Petersen J, Batsberg W, Larsen E (1990) Contact dermatitis from Naphthol AS. Contact Dermatitis 22:161–163

299. Neomycin (Neomycin B Hydrochloride, Neomycin B Sulfate)

Framycetin, Soframycin®

CAS Registry Number [1404–04–2] (CAS Registry Number [25389–99–5],
CAS Registry Number [1405–10–3])

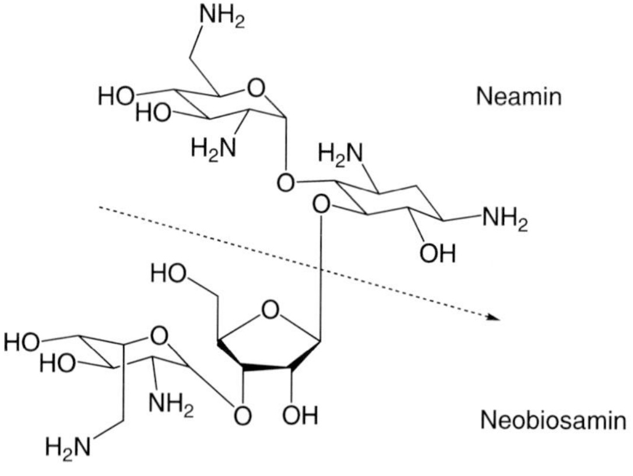

Neomycin is an antibiotic complex of the aminoglycosides group, extracted from *Streptomyces fradiae*. It is composed of neomycin A (neamin) and an isomer neobiosamin, either neomycin B (framycetin or Soframycin®) or neomycin C. Its use has been progressively forbidden in cosmetics and as an additive for animal feed. Occupational contact dermatitis occurs in workers at animal feed mills, in veterinaries or in health workers. Nonoccupational dermatitis mainly concerns patients with chronic dermatitis, leg ulcers or chronic otitis. Cross-sensitivity is usual with other amino-glycosides (amikacin, arbekacin, butirosin, dibekacin, gentamicin, isepamicin, kanamycin, paromomycin, ribostamycin, sisomycin, tobramycin), is rare with netilmicin and streptomycin, but non-existent with spectinomycin.

Suggested Reading

Le Coz CJ (2001) Fiche d'éviction en cas d'hypersensibilité à la néomycine. Ann Dermatol Venereol 128 : 1359–1360

Mancuso G, Staffa M, Errani A, Berdondini RM, Fabri P (1990) Occupational dermatitis in animal feed mill workers. Contact Dermatitis 22 : 37–41

Rebandel P, Rudzki E (1986) Occupational contact sensitivity in oculists. Contact Dermatitis 15 : 92

300. Nicotine

CAS Registry Number [55–11–5]

Nicotine is an alkaloid found in tobacco, and is responsible for its pharmacological effects and addiction. Contact dermatitis from nicotine, considered as rare, has been more frequent since its use in transdermal systems. Irritant dermatitis is mainly encountered, as contact urticaria seems to be rare. Allergic contact dermatitis, sometimes generalized, has been reported, with positive patch testing to nicotine base (10% ethanol or petrolatum). No conse-quences have been reported in patients who start smoking again after skin sensitization.

Suggested Reading

Bircher AJ, Howald H, Rufli T (1991) Adverse skin reactions to nicotine in a transdermal therapeutic system. Contact Dermatitis 25 : 230–236

Vincenzi C, Tosti A, Cirone M, Guarrera M, Cusano F (1993) Allergic con-tact dermatitis from transdermal nicotine systems. Contact Dermatitis 29 : 104–105

301. 3-Nitro-4-Hydroxyethylaminophenol

4-[(2-Hydroxyethyl)Amino]-3-Nitrophenol

CAS Registry Number [65235–31–6]

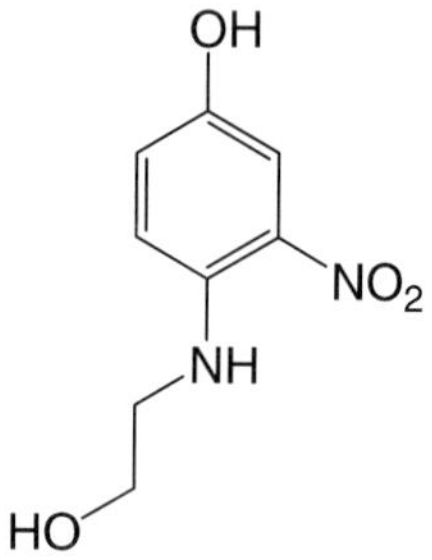

This dye belongs to the aminophenol class and is used as a hair colorant, particularly in semi-permanent hair dye preparations.

Suggested Reading

Le Coz CJ, Kühne S, Engel F (2003) Hair dye allergy due to 3-nitro-*p*-hydroxyethyl-aminophenol. Contact Dermatitis 49:103

302. 2-Nitro-4-Phenylenediamine

o-Nitro-*p*-Phenylenediamine, ONPD, CI 76070

CAS Registry Number [5307–14–2]

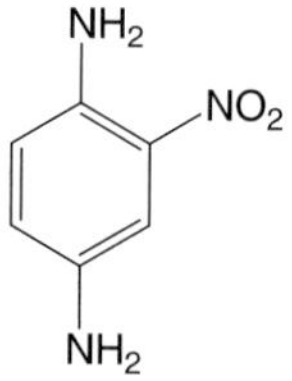

ONPD is a hair dye and a sensitizer in hairdressers and consumers who are generally sensitive to PPD too.

Suggested Reading

Frosch PJ, Burrows D, Camarasa JG, Dooms-Goossens A, Ducombs G, Lahti A, Menné T, Rycroft RJG, Shaw S, White IR, Wilkinson JD (1993) Allergic reactions to a hairdresser's series: results from 9 European centres. Contact Dermatitis 28:180–183

Guerra L, Tosti A, Bardazzi F, Pigatto P, Lisi P, Santucci B, Valsecchi R, Schena D, Angelini G, Sertoli A, Ayala F, Kokelj F (1992) Contact dermatitis in hairdressers: the Italian experience. Gruppo Italiano Ricerca Dermatiti da Contatto e Ambientali. Contact Dermatitis 26:101–107

Van der Walle HB, Brunsveld VM (1994) Dermatitis in hairdressers (I). The experience of the past 4 years. Contact Dermatitis 30:217–220

303. Nitrofurazone

Nitrofural, Nitrozone, Aldomycin

CAS Registry Numbers [59–87–0], [60051–85–6], [8027–71–2]

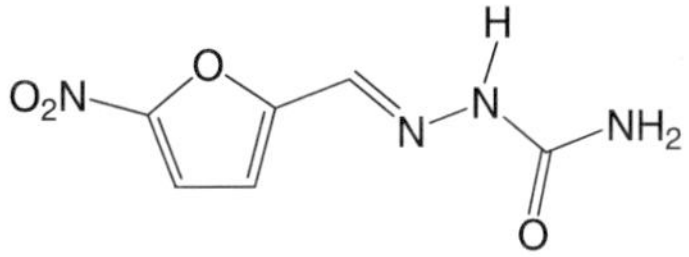

Nitrofurazone is an antibacterial agent used in animal feeds. Occupational dermatitis was reported in cattle breeders or farmers.

Suggested Reading

Condé-Salazar L, Guimaraens D, Gonzalez MA, Molina A (1995) Occupational allergic contact dermatitis from nitrofurazone. Contact Dermatitis 32:307–308

Vilaplana J, Grimalt F, Romaguera C (1990) Contact dermatitis from furaltadone in animal feed. Contact Dermatitis 22:232–233

304. Nitroglycerin

Glyceryl Trinitrate, Glycerol Trinitrate

CAS Registry Number [55–63–0]

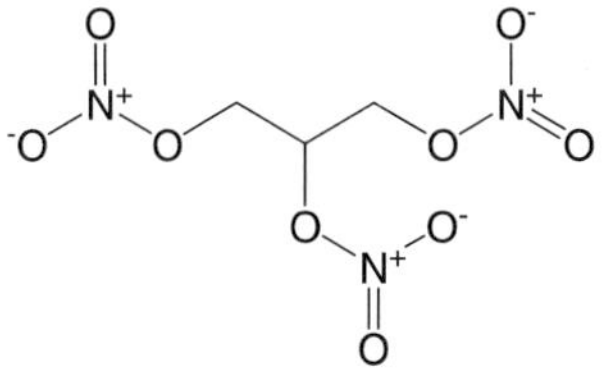

Nitroglycerin is an explosive agent contained in dynamite, and an antianginal and vasodilator treatment available in systemic and topical forms. It is a well known irritant agent in dynamite manufacture. It can also cause allergic reactions in employees of explosives manufacturers, and in the pharmaceutical industry. Transdermal systems are the main source of iatrogenic sensitization. Nitroglycerin can cross-react with isosorbide dinitrate.

Suggested Reading

Aquilina S, Felice H, Boffa MJ (2002) Allergic reactions to glyceryl trinitrate and isosorbide dinitrate demonstrating cross-sensitivity. Clin Exp Dermatol 27:700–702

Kanerva L, Laine R, Jolanki R, Tarvainen K, Estlander T, Helander I (1991) Occupational allergic contact dermatitis caused by nitroglycerin. Contact Dermatitis 24:356–362

Machet L, Martin L, Toledano C, Jan V, Lorette G, Vaillant L (1999) Allergic contact dermatitis from nitroglycerin contained in 2 transdermal systems. Dermatology 198:106–107

305. Nonoxynols

Nonylphenol Ethoxylates, PEG-(n) Nonyl Phenyl Ether, Polyoxyethylene (n) Nonyl Phenyl Ether

CAS Registry Number [26027–38–3] and more than 25 other numbers

Their general formula is $C_9H_{19}C_6H_4(OCH_2CH_2)_nOH$. Each nonoxynol is characterized by the number (n) of ethylene oxide units repeated in the chain; for example, nonoxynol-9, nonoxynol-14. They are present in detergents, liquid soaps, emulsifiers for creams, fabric softeners, photographic paper additives, hair dyes, lubricating oils, spermicides, and anti-infective agents. They are irritants and sensitizers. Nonoxynol-6 was reported as a sensitizing agent in an industrial hand cleanser and in a crack-indicating fluid in the metal industry. Nonoxynol-9 is the most commonly used, as a preservative in topical antiseptics or in spermicides, acting as a iodophor in PVP-iodine solutions. Nonoxynol-10 was reported as a UVB-photosensitizer. Nonoxynol-12 caused contact dermatitis in a domestic cleaner who used a polish containing it.

Suggested Reading

Dooms-Goossens A, Deveylder H, de Alam AG, Lachapelle JM, Tennstedt D, Degreef H (1989) Contact sensitivity to nonoxynols as a cause of intolerance to antiseptic preparations. J Am Acad Dermatol 21:723–727

Meding B (1985) Occupational contact dermatitis from nonylphenolpoly-glycolether. Contact Dermatitis 13:122–123

Nethercott JR, Lawrence MJ (1984) Allergic contact dermatitis due to nonylphenol ethoxylate (nonoxynol-6). Contact Dermatitis 10:235–239

Wilkinson SM, Beck MH, August PJ (1995) Allergic contact dermatitis from nonoxynol-12 in a polish. Contact Dermatitis 33:128–129

306. Octocrylene

Octocrilene

CAS Registry Number [6197–30–4]

Octocrylene is an anti-UVB filter used in cosmetics that may induce photoallergic contact dermatitis.

Suggested Reading

Carrotte-Lefebvre I, Bonnevalle A, Segard M, Delaporte E, Thomas P (2003) Contact allergy to octocrylene. Contact Dermatitis 48:46–47

307. Octyl Gallate

CAS Registry Number
[1034–01–1]

Octyl gallate, a gallate ester (E 311), is an antioxidant added to foods and cosmetics to prevent oxidation of unsaturated fatty acids. Cases were sparsely reported in food industry or from lipsticks. Patch tests are frequently irritant.

Suggested Reading

De Groot AC, Gerkens F (1990) Occupational airborne contact dermatitis from octyl gallate. Contact Dermatitis 23:184–186

Giordano-Labadie F, Schwarze HP, Bazex J (2000) Allergic contact dermatitis from octyl gallate in lipstick. Contact Dermatitis 42:51

308. 2-n-Octyl-4-Isothiazolin-3-one

Kathon® LM, Kathon® 4200, Kathon® 893, Pancil, Skane M-8

CAS Registry Number
[26530–20–1]

This isothiazolinone, contained in relatively few products compared to other isothiazolinones, is used in cleaning and polishing agents, latex paints, stains, adhesives, wood and leather preservatives, metalworking fluids (cutting oils), and plastic manufacture.

Suggested Reading

Oleaga JM, Aguirre A, Landa N, Gonzalez M, Diaz-Perez JL (1992) Allergic contact dermatitis from Kathon 893. Contact Dermatitis 27:345–346

Young HS, Ferguson JEF, Beck MH (2004) Contact dermatitis from 2-n-octyl-4-isothiazoline-3-one in a PhD student. Contact Dermatitis 50:47–48

309. Olaquindox

N-(2-Hydroxyethyl)-3-Methyl-2-Quinoxalinecarboxamide 1,4-Dioxide

CAS Registry Number
[23696–28–8]

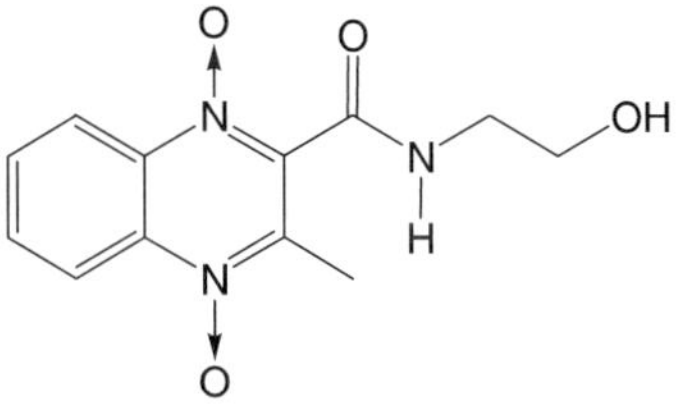

Olaquindox is an antibacterial agent derivative of quinoxaline, used as a growth promoter of pigs. It can be found in Bayo-N-Ox® and Proquindox® and numerous other pig feeds. It is a photosensitizer that forms reactive photoproducts on light exposure. It can induce photoallergic contact dermatitis and persistent light reactions.

Suggested Reading

Belhadjali H, Marguery MC, Journe F, Giordano-Labadie F, Lefebvre H, Bazex J (2002) Allergic and photoallergic contact dermatitis to Olaquindox in a pig breeder with prolonged photosensitivity. Photodermatol Photoimmunol Photomed 18:52–53

Kumar A, Freeman S (1996) Photoallergic contact dermatitis in a pig farmer caused by olaquindox. Contact Dermatitis 35:249–250

Schauder S, Schröder W, Geier J (1996) Olaquindox-induced airborne photoallergic contact dermatitis followed by transient or persistent light reactions in 15 pig breeders. Contact Dermatitis 35:344–354

310. Oxacillin

CAS Registry Number: [66–79–5]

Oxacillin Sodium Salt Monohydrate

CAS Registry Number: [7240–38–2]

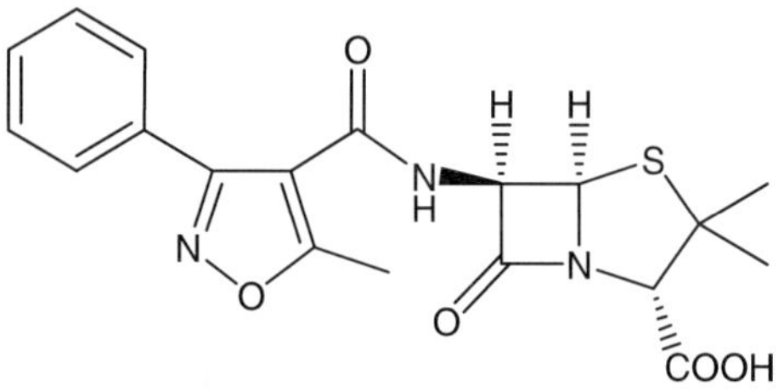

Oxacillin is a semi-synthetic penicillin of the group M. It is closely related to cloxacillin.

Suggested Reading
Budavari S, O'Neil MJ, Smith A, Heckelman PE, Kinneary JF (eds) (1996) The Merck Index, 12th edn. Merck, Whitehouse Station, N.J., USA

311. 7-Oxodehydroabietic Acid

CAS Registry Number [18684–55–4]

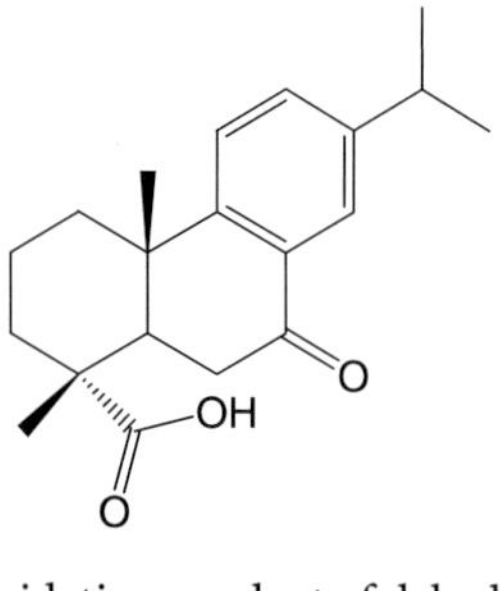

7-Oxodehydroabietic acid is an auto-oxidation product of dehydroabietic acid, and an allergen contained in colophony.

Suggested Reading
Bergh M, Menné T, Karlberg AT (1994) Colophony in paper-based surgical clothing. Contact Dermatitis 31:332–333

312. Oxprenolol

CAS Registry Number [6452–71–7]

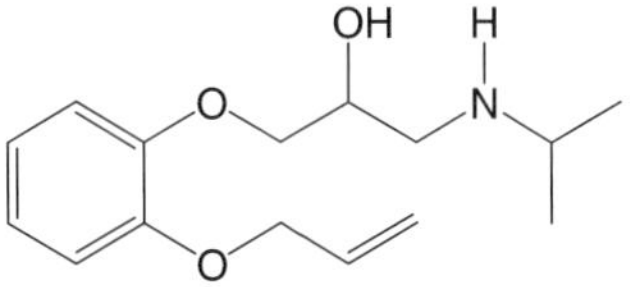

The beta-blocker oxprenolol induced contact dermatitis in a worker at a pharmaceutical plant, in a division for drug synthesis. Epichlorhydrin was also used for the production of drugs propranolol and oxprenolol.

Suggested Reading

Rebandel P, Rudzki E (1990) Dermatitis caused by epichlorhydrin, oxprenolol hydrochloride and propranolol hydrochloride. Contact Dermatitis 23:199

313. Pantothenol

2,4-Dihydroxy-*N*-(3-Hydroxypropyl)-3,3-Dimethylbutanamide, Pantothenylol, *N*-Pantoyl-3-Propanolamine, Panthenol, Pantothenyl Alcohol

CAS Registry Number [81–13–0]

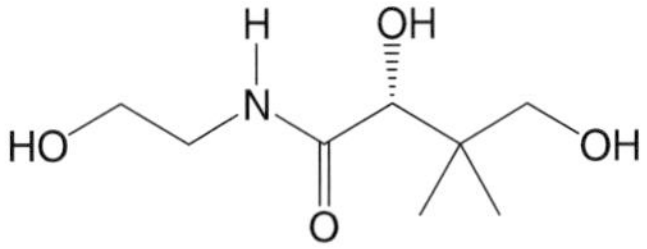

Pan(to)thenol is the alcohol corresponding to pantothenic acid, of the vitamin B5 group. It is used as a food additive, and in skin and hair products as a conditioning agent. Contact dermatitis and urticaria have been reported.

Suggested Reading

Schalock PC, Storrs FJ, Morrison L (2000) Contact urticaria from panthenol in hair conditioner. Contact Dermatitis 43:223

Stables GI, Wilkinson SM (1998) Allergic contact dermatitis due to panthenol. Contact Dermatitis 38:236–237

314. Parabens (Parahydroxybenzoic Acid Esters)

Methylparaben, E218, E219 (Sodium Salt)

CAS Registry Number [99–76–3], E219 (Sodium Salt), CAS Registry Number [5026–62–0]

Ethylparaben, E214, E215 (Sodium Salt)

CAS Registry Number [120–47–8]. E215 (Sodium Salt), CAS Registry Number [35285–68–8]

Propylparaben, E216, E217 (Sodium Salt)

CAS Registry Number [94–13–3], E217 (Sodium Salt), CAS Registry Number [35285–69–9]

Isopropylparaben

CAS Registry Number [4191–73–5]

Butylparaben

CAS Registry Number [94–26–8]

Isobutylparaben

CAS Registry Number [4247–02–3]

Phenylparaben

CAS Registry Number [17696–62–7]

Benzylparaben

CAS Registry Number [94–18–8]

Phenoxyethylparaben

CAS Registry Number [55468–88–7]

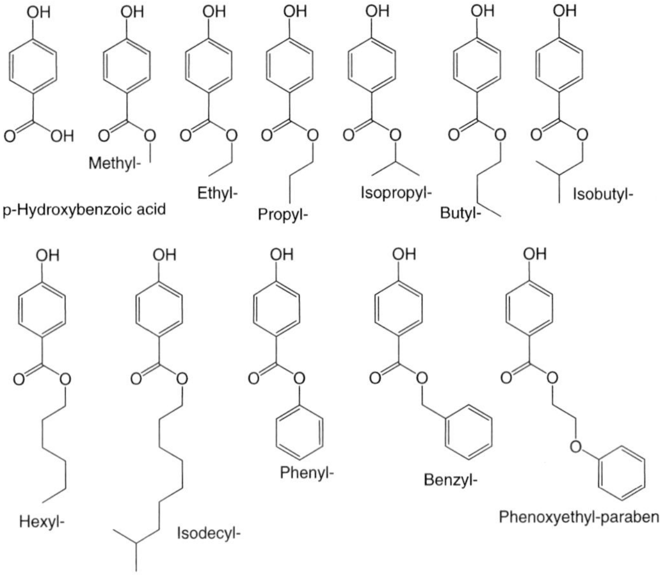

Parabens are esters formed by *p*-hydroxybenzoic acid and an alcohol. They are largely used as biocides in cosmetics and toiletries, medicaments, or food. They have synergistic power with other biocides. Parabens can induce allergic contact dermatitis, mainly in chronic dermatitis and wounded skin.

Suggested Reading

Le Coz CJ (2004) Fiche d'éviction en cas d'hypersensibilité aux esters de l'acide *para*-hydroxybenzoïque (parahydroxybenzoates ou parabens). Ann Dermatol Venereol 131:309–310

315. Paraphenylenediamine

PPD, *p*-Phenylenediamine, 4-Phenylenediamine

CAS Registry Number [106–50–3]

PPD is a colorless compound oxidized by hydrogen peroxide in the presence of ammonia. It is then polymerized to a color by a coupling agent. Although a well-known allergen in hair dyes, PPD can be found as a cause of contact dermatitis in chin rest stains or in milk testers. It is also a marker of group sensitivity to *para* amino compounds such as benzocaine, some azo-dyes and some previous antibacterial sulphonamides.

Suggested Reading

Bork K (1993) Allergic contact dermatitis on a violinist's neck from para-phenylenediamine in a chin rest stain. Contact Dermatitis 28:250–251

Frosch PJ, Burrows D, Camarasa JG, Dooms-Goossens A, Ducombs G, Lahti A, Menné T, Rycroft RJG, Shaw S, White IR, Wilkinson JD (1993) Allergic reactions to a hairdresser's series: results from 9 European centres. Contact Dermatitis 28:180–183

Guerra L, Tosti A, Bardazzi F, Pigatto P, Lisi P, Santucci B, Valsecchi R, Schena D, Angelini G, Sertoli A, Ayala F, Kokelj F (1992) Contact dermatitis in hairdressers: the Italian experience. Gruppo Italiano Ricerca Dermatiti da Contatto e Ambientali. Contact Dermatitis 26:101–107

Le Coz CJ, Lefebvre C, Keller F, Grosshans E (2000) Allergic contact dermatitis caused by skin painting (pseudotattooing) with black henna, a mixture of henna and *p*-phenylenediamine and its derivatives. Arch Dermatol 136:1515–1517

Rebandel P, Rudzki E (1995) Occupational allergy to *p*-phenylenediamine in milk testers. Contact Dermatitis 33:138

316. Paraquat (Dichloride, Methosulfate)

1-1'-Dimethyl-4,4'-Bipyridinium Salt

CAS Registry Numbers [4685–14–7], [116047–10–0]
(CAS Registry Number [1910–42–5],
CAS Registry Number [2074–50–2])

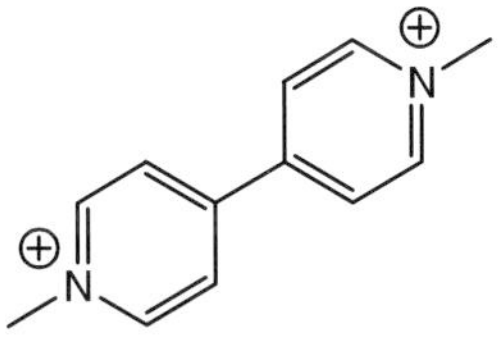

Paraquat is a quaternary ammonium compound with herbicide properties, as diquat. It is contained in Cekuquat® or Dipril®. It can cause contact and phototoxic contact dermatitis, acne, and leukoderma mainly in agricultural workers.

Suggested Reading

Vilaplana J, Azon A, Romaguera C, Lecha M (1993) Phototoxic contact dermatitis with toxic hepatitis due to the percutaneous absorption of paraquat. Contact Dermatitis 29 : 163–164

317. Parathion

Parathion-Ethyl: Parathion, Ethylparathion, Corothion, Dantion, Folidol

CAS Registry Number [56–38–2]

Paration-Methyl: Methylparathion, Matafos, Paratox, Folidol M

CAS Registry Number [298–00–0]

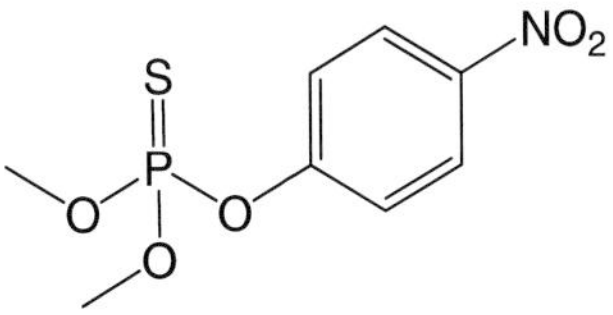

Methyl-Parathion

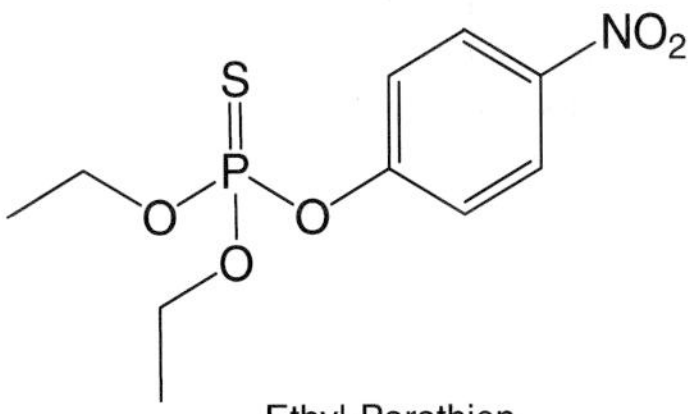

Ethyl-Parathion

One case was reported of a bullous contact dermatitis due to ethyl-parathion. A case of sensitization to methyl-parathion was described in a female agricultural worker with multiple sensitization.

Suggested Reading

Jung HD, Holzegel K (1988) Akute Toxisch-bullöse Kontaktdermatitis durch den Phosphorsäurester Parathionethyl im Follidel-Öl. Aktuel Dermatol 14:19–31

Pevny I (1980) Pestizid-Allergie. Dermatosen 28:186–189

318. Parthenolide

CAS Registry Number [20554–84–1]

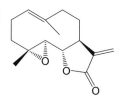

Parthenolide is a sesquiterpene lactone found Asteraceae–Compositae such as feverfew (*Tanacetum parthenium* Schultz-Bip.) or congress grass (*Parthenium hysterophorus* L.).

Suggested Reading

Hausen BM, Osmundsen PE (1983) Contact allergy to parthenolide in *Tanacetum parthenium* (L.) Schultz-Bip. (feverfew, Asteraceae) and cross-reactions to related sesquiterpene lactone containing Compositae species. Acta Derm Venereol (Stockh) 63:308–314

Lamminpää A, Estlander T, Jolanki R, Kanerva L (1996) Occupational allergic contact dermatitis caused by decorative plants. Contact Dermatitis 34:330–335

Paulsen E, Andersen KE, Hausen BM (1993) Compositae dermatitis in a Danish dermatology department in one year (I). Results of routine patch testing with the sesquiterpene lactone mix supplemented with aimed patch testing with extracts and sesquiterpene lactones of Compositae plants. Contact Dermatitis 29:6–10

319. Penicillins

CAS Registry Number [1406–05–9]

for penicillin

Penicillins can induce contact dermatitis, contact urticaria, and systemic and sometimes severe reactions. Occupational sensitivity to penicillins concerns health workers, workers in the pharmaceutical industry and veterinaries, since these antibiotics are used by veterinarians and cattle breeders as medications and animal feed antibiotic. All penicillins contain the 6-aminopenicillanic acid moiety. Penicillins of G, V, A, and M groups are characterized by a specific C_7 side chain. Cross-reactivity is possible between several penicillins but is not systematic since both immediate- and delayed-type sensitivity can implicate the 6-aminopenicillanic acid moiety, or be specific to the 7-side-chain.

Suggested Reading

Guerra L, Venturo N, Tardio M, Tosti A (1995) Airborne contact dermatitis from animal feed antibiotics. Contact Dermatitis 32: 61–62

Rudzki E, Rebandel P, Grzywa Z (1989) Patch tests with occupational contactants in nurses, doctors and dentists. Contact Dermatitis 20: 247–250

320. Pentachloronitrobenzene

Quintozene, PCNB, Brassicol, Terrachlor®

CAS Registry Number [82–68–8]

Pentachloronitrobenzene is a pesticide and a fungicide. Sensitization can occur in farmers or in chemical plants.

Suggested Reading

O'Malley M, Rodriguez P, Maibach HI (1995) Pesticide patch testing: California nursery workers and controls. Contact Dermatitis 32:61–62

Sharma VK, Kaur S (1990) Contact sensitization by pesticides in farmers. Contact Dermatitis 23:77–80

321. Pentadecylcatechol

3-Pentadecylcatechol, Hydrourushiol, Tetrahydrourushiol

CAS Registry Number [492–89–7]

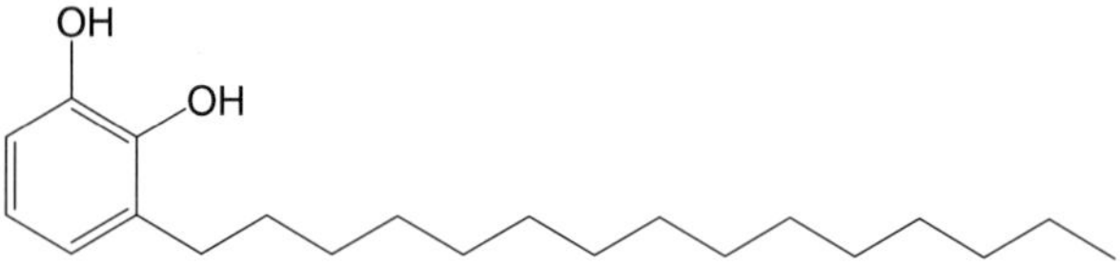

Pentadecylcatechol belongs to the urushiols, and is the main allergen of the Anacardiaceae poison ivy (*Toxicodendron radicans*) and of Poison oak (*Toxicodendron diversiloba, Rhus diversiloba*).

Suggested Reading

Epstein WL (1994) Occupational poison ivy and oak dermatitis. Dermatol Clin 12:511–516

322. Phenoxyethanol

2-Phenoxyethanol

CAS Registry Numbers [122–99–6], [37220–49–8], [56257–90–0]

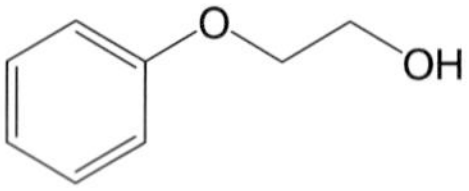

Phenoxyethanol is an aromatic ether-alcohol used mainly as a preservative, mostly with methyldibromoglutaronitrile (in Euxyl®

K 400) or with parabens. Sensitization to this molecule is very rare.

Suggested Reading

Vigan M, Brechat N, Girardin P, Adessi B, Meyer JP, Vuitton D, Laurent R (1996) Un nouvel allergène: le dibromodicyanobutane. Etude sur 310 patients de janvier à décembre 1994. Ann Dermatol Venereol 123: 322–324

323. Phenyl Glycidyl Ether

CAS Registry Numbers [122–60–1], [66527–93–3]

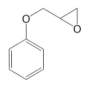

This monoglycidyl derivative is a reactive diluent in epoxy resins Bisphenol A type. It is a component of epoxy paints, epoxy glues, and epoxy resins. Sensitization has been observed in many professions, such as in construction workers, marble workers, ceramic workers, and shoemakers.

Suggested Reading

Angelini G, Rigano L, Foti C, Grandolfo M, Vena GA, Bonamonte D, Soleo L, Scorpiniti AA (1996) Occupational sensitization to epoxy resin and reactive diluents in marble workers. Contact Dermatitis 35:11–16

Condé-Salazar L, Gonzalez de Domingo MA, Guimaraens D (1994) Sensitization to epoxy resin systems in special flooring workers. Contact Dermatitis 31:157–160

Jolanki R, Kanerva L, Estlander T, Tarvainen K, Keskinen H, Henriks-Eckerman ML (1990) Occupational dermatoses from epoxy resin compounds. Contact Dermatitis 23:172–183

Mancuso G, Reggiani M, Berdondini RM (1996) Occupational dermatitis in shoemakers. Contact Dermatitis 34:17–22

Seidenari S, Danese P, di Nardo A, Manzini BM, Motolese A (1990) Contact sensitization among ceramics workers. Contact Dermatitis 22:45–49

Tarvainen K (1995) Analysis of patients with allergic patch test reactions to a plastic and glues series. Contact Dermatitis 32:346–351

324. Phenyl-Alpha-Naphthylamine

Neozone A, CI 44050

CAS Registry Number [90–30–2]

Phenyl-alpha-naphthylamine is contained in some rubbers and oils as an antioxidant of the amine group. It is closely related to phenyl-beta-naphthylamine and to di-beta-naphthyl-*p*-phenylenediamine, but without cross-reactivity.

Suggested Reading

Carmichael AJ, Foulds IS (1990) Isolated naphthylamine allergy to phenyl-alpha-naphthylamine. Contact Dermatitis 22:298–299

Svedman C, Isaksson M, Zimerson E, Bruze M (2004) Occupational contact dermatitis from a grease. Dermatitis 15:41–44

325. Phenyl-Beta-Naphthylamine

N-Phenyl-2-Naphthylamine, Neozone

CAS Registry Numbers [135–88–6], [52907–17–2], [84420–28–0]

Phenyl-beta-naphthylamine is an amine compound. Sensitization was reported in patients with hypersensitivity from rubber.

Suggested Reading

Condé-Salazar L, Guimaraens D, Romero LV, Gonzalez MA (1987) Unusual allergic contact dermatitis to aromatic amines. Contact Dermatitis 17:42–44

Condé-Salazar L, Del-Rio E, Guimaraens D, Gonzalez Domingo A (1993) Type IV allergy to rubber additives: a 10-year study of 686 cases. J Am Acad Dermatol 29:176–180

Kiec-Swierczynska M (1995) Occupational sensitivity to rubber. Contact
    Dermatitis 32:171–172

326. Phenylephrine (Hydrochloride)

CAS Registry Number [59–42–7]

Phenylephrine Hydrochloride

CAS Registry Number [61–76–7]

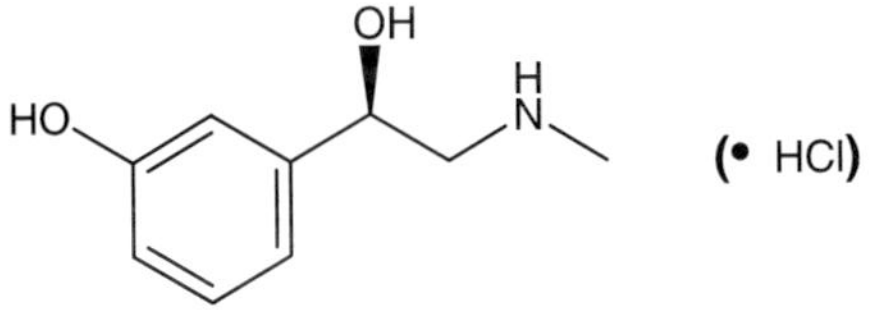

Phenylephrine hydrochloride is an alpha-adrenergic agonist, used
as a mydriatic and decongestant in eyedrops.

Suggested Reading
Narayan S, Prais L, Foulds IS (2002) Allergic contact dermatitis caused by
    phenylephrine eyedrops. Am J Contact Dermat 13:208–209

327. Phenylethyl Caffeate

Caffeic Acid Phenethyl Ester, Capee

CAS Registry Number [104594–70–9]

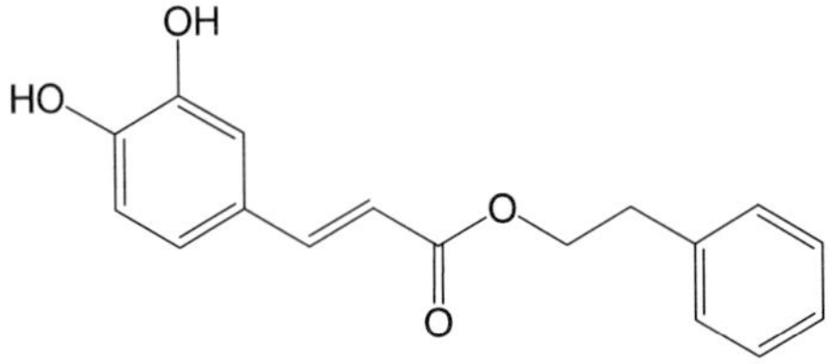

Capee is one of the allergens of propolis (bee glue). It is also contained in poplar bud secretions.

Suggested Reading

Lamminpää A, Estlander T, Jolanki R, Kanerva L (1996) Occupational allergic contact dermatitis caused by decorative plants. Contact Dermatitis 34:330–335

Oliwiecki S, Beck MH, Hausen BM (1992) Occupational contact dermatitis from caffeates in poplar bud resin in a tree surgeon. Contact Dermatitis 27:127–128

328. Phthalic Anhydride

CAS Registry Numbers
[85–44–9], [39363–63–8]

Phthalic anhydride is used in the manufacture of unsaturated polyesters and as a curing agent for epoxy resins. When used as a pigment, it can be responsible for sensitization in ceramic workers. Phthalic anhydride per se is not responsible for the sensitization to the resin used in nail varnishes phthalic anhydride/trimellitic anhydride/glycols copolymer, CAS Registry Number [85–44–9].

Suggested Reading

Seidenari S, Danese P, di Nardo A, Manzini BM, Motolese A (19909 Contact sensitization among ceramics workers. Contact Dermatitis 22:45–49

Tarvainen K, Jolanki R, Estlander T, Tupasela O, Pfäffli P, Kanerva L (1995) Immunologic contact urticaria due to airborne methylhexahydrophthalic and methyltetrahydrophthalic anhydrides. Contact Dermatitis 32:204–209

329. Picric Acid

CI 10305

CAS Registry Number
[88–89–1]

Contact dermatitis occurred primarily in the explosives industry.

Suggested Reading

Aguirre A, Sanz de Galdeano C, Oleaga JM, Eizaguirre X, Diaz Perez JL (1993) Allergic contact dermatitis from picric acid. Contact Dermatitis 28:291

Hausen BM (1994) Letter to the editor. Picric acid. Contact Dermatitis 30:59

330. Alpha-Pinene

CAS Registry Numbers [80–56–8], [2437–95–8]

Alpha-pinene is the major constituent of turpentine (about 80%). It exists in levogyre form in European turpentine, and in dextrogyre form in turpentine found in North-Americans. Sensitization occurs mainly in painters, polishers, and varnishers, and in those in the perfume and in the ceramics industry.

Suggested Reading

Lear JT, Heagerty AHM, Tan BB, Smith AG, English JSC (1996) Transient re-emergence of oil turpentine allergy in the pottery industry. Contact Dermatitis 35:169–172

Moura C, Dias M, Vale T (1994) Contact dermatitis in painters, polishers and varnishers. Contact Dermatitis 31:51–53

331. Beta-Pinene

Nopinene, Terebenthene

CAS Registry Number [127–91–3]

Beta-pinene is a component of turpentine. Concentrations vary with the source, and seem higher in European (Portuguese) than in Asian (Indonesian) turpentine.

Suggested Reading

Lear JT, Heagerty AHM, Tan BB, Smith AG, English JSC (1996) Transient
   re-emergence of oil turpentine allergy in the pottery industry. Contact
   Dermatitis 35:169–172

332. Piperazine

Diethylenediamine

CAS Registry Number [110–85–0]

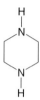

Piperazine is contained in pyrazinobutazone, an equimolar salt of
piperazine and phenylbutazone. Among occupational cases, most
were reported in the pharmaceutical industry or laboratory workers, in nurses, and in veterinarians.

Suggested Reading

Dorado Bris JM, Montanes Aragues M, Sols Candela M, Garcia Diez A
   (1992) Contact sensitivity to pyrazinobutazone (Carudol®) with positive oral provocation test. Contact Dermatitis 26:355–356
Rudzki E, Rebandel P, Grzywa Z, Pomorski Z, Jakiminska B, Zawisza E
   (1982) Occupational dermatitis in veterinarians. Contact Dermatitis
   8:72–73

333. Piroxicam

CAS Registry Number [36332–90–4]

This nonsteroidal anti-inflammatory drug belongs to the oxicam
class. It induces photo-allergic contact dermatitis rather than contact allergy. Systemic photosensitivity is frequent, in patients prev-

iously sensitized to thiomersal. Thiosalicylic acid, the nonmer-
curial moiety of thiomersal, is a marker of photoallergy to piroxicam. Reactions are expected with piroxicam β-cyclodextrin but
cross-sensitivity is generally not observed to tenoxicam or melox-
icam (personal observations).

Suggested Reading

Arévalo A, Blancas R, Ancona A (1995) Occupational contact dermatitis
     from piroxicam. Am J Contact Dermat 6:113–114
De la Cuadra J, Pujol C, Aliaga A (1989) Clinical evidence of cross-sensi-
     tivity between thiosalicylic acid, a contact allergen, and piroxicam, a
     photoallergen. Contact Dermatitis 21:349–351

334. Pivampicillin

CAS Registry Number [33817–20–8]

Pivampicillin Hydrochloride

CAS Registry Number [26309–95–5]

Pivampicillin is a prodrug of ampicillin. It caused sensitization in
56 workers at a penicillin factory. Pivampicillin and pivmecillinam
were responsible for contact dermatitis in pharmaceutical
production workers. Ampicillin, mecillinam or amdinocillin,
penicillin V and penicillin G were also implicated in cross-reactions.

Suggested Reading

Moller NE, von Würden K (1992) Hypersensitivity to semisynthetic peni-
     cillins and cross-reactivity with penicillin. Contact Dermatitis 26:
     351–352
Moller NE, Nielsen B, von Würden K (1990) Changes in penicillin contam-
     ination and allergy in factory workers. Contact Dermatitis 22:106–107

335. Potassium Metabisulfite

Sodium Pyrosulfite, Disodium Disulfite, E224

CAS Registry Number
[16731–55–8]

Potassium metabisulfite is an antioxidant used as an antifermentative agent in breweries and wineries, as a preservative of fruits and vegetables, and to bleach straw. Reactions to both sodium and potassium metabisulfite are expected.

Suggested Reading

Budavari S, O'Neil MJ, Smith A, Heckelman PE, Kinneary JF (eds) (1996) The Merck Index, 12th edn. Merck, Whitehouse Station, N.J., USA

336. Povidone-Iodine

Polyvinylpyrrolidone-Iodine, PVP-Iodine

CAS Registry Number
[25655–41–8]

Povidone-iodine is iodophor, used as a topical antiseptic. A 10% povidone-iodine solution contains 1% available iodine, but free-iodine is at 0.1% concentration. Skin exposure causes irritant rather than allergic contact dermatitis. In such a situation however, iodine seems to be the true hapten.

Suggested Reading

Lachapelle JM (2005) Allergic contact dermatitis from povidone-iodine: a re-evaluation study. Contact Dermatitis 52:9–10

Tosti A, Vincenzi C, Bardazzi F, Mariani R (1990) Allergic contact dermatitis due to povidoneiodine. Contact Dermatitis 23:197–198

337. Prilocaine (Hydrochloride)

CAS Registry Number [25655–41–8] (CAS Registry Number [1786–81–8])

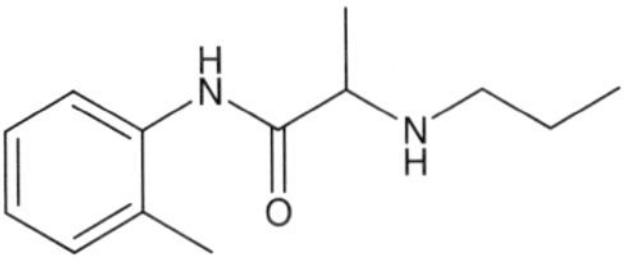

Prilocaine in a local anesthetic of the amide group. It can induce allergic contact dermatitis, particularly from EMLA® cream.

Suggested Reading

Le Coz CJ, Cribier BJ, Heid E (1996) Patch testing in suspected allergic contact dermatitis due to Emla® cream in haemodialyzed patients. Contact Dermatitis 35:316–317

338. Primin

CAS Registry Number [15121–94–5]

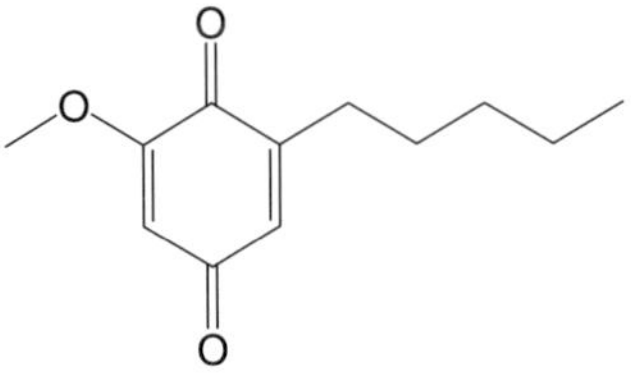

Primin is the major allergen of *Primula obconica* Hance (Primulaceae family). Allergic contact dermatitis is mainly occupational, occurring in florists and horticulturists.

Suggested Reading

Christensen LP, Larsen E (2000) Direct emission of the allergen primin from intact *Primula obconica* plants. Contact Dermatitis 42:149–153

Lamminpää A, Estlander T, Jolanki R, Kanerva L (1996) Occupational allergic contact dermatitis caused by decorative plants. Contact Dermatitis 34:330–335

339. Pristinamycin

Pristinamycin

CAS Registry Number [270076–60–3]

Pristinamycin IA (Streptogramin B, Mikamycin IA, Ostreogrycin B, Vernamycin B$_{alpha}$)

CAS Registry Number [3131–03–1]

Pristinamycin IIA (Mikamycin A, Ostreogrycin A, Pristinamycin II$_A$, Staphylomycin M$_1$, Streptogramin A, Vernamycin A, Virginiamycin M$_1$)

CAS Registry Number [21411–53–0]

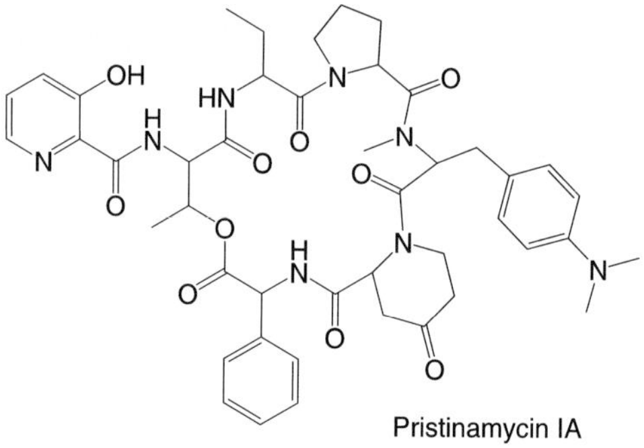

Pristinamycin IA

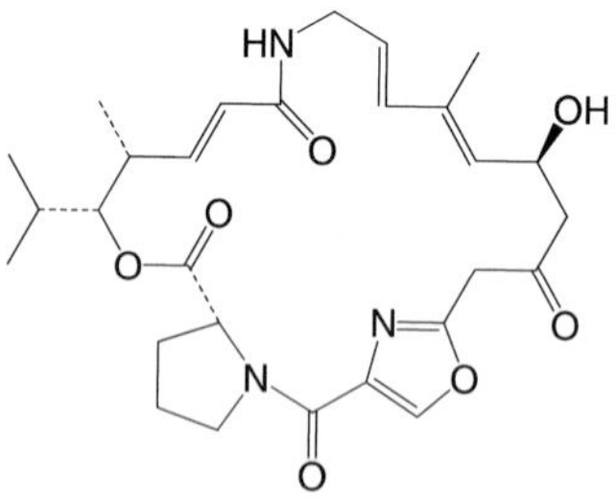

Pristinamycin IIA

Pristinamycin is a systemic antibiotic of the synergistins/strepto-gramins class, composed of two subunits: pristinamycin IA and pristinamycin IIA. It induces several types of drug reactions such as maculo-papular exanthema, systemic dermatitis or acute gener-alized exanthematous pustulosis. Some patients have been prev-iously skin-sensitized by virginiamycin (see below). Cross-reac-tivity is expected to virginiamycin CAS [11006–76–1] and to the associated dalfopristin (CAS [112362–50–2]) and quinupristin (CAS [120138–50–3]).

Suggested Reading
Barbaud A, Trechot P, Weber-Muller F, Ulrich G, Commun N, Schmutz JL (2004) Drug skin tests in cutaneous adverse drug reactions to pristi-namycin: 29 cases with a study of cross-reactions between synergis-tins. Contact Dermatitis 50 : 22–26

340. Procaine (Hydrochloride)

2-Diethylaminoethyl 4-Aminobenzoate, Novocaine®

CAS Registry Number [59–46–1]

Procaine Hydrochloride

CAS Registry Number [51–05–8]

Procaine is a local anesthetic with *para*-amino function. Sensitiza-tion mainly concerns the medical, dental, and veterinary profes-sions.

Suggested Reading
Berova N, Stranky L, Krasteva M (1990) Studies on contact dermatitis in stomatological staff. Dermatol Monatschr 176 : 15–18
Rudzki E, Rebandel P, Grzywa Z, Pomorski Z, Jakiminska B, Zawisza E (1982) Occupational dermatitis in veterinarians. Contact Dermatitis 8 : 72–73

341. Propacetamol

4-Acetamidophenyl *N,N*-Diethylglycinate Hydrochloride

CAS Registry Number
[66532–85–2]

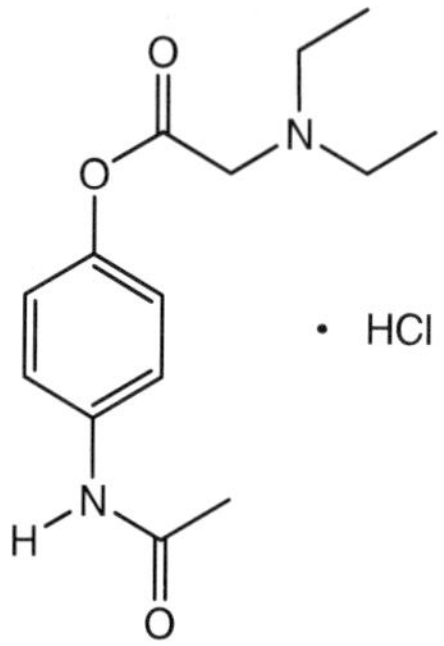

Propacetamol is a prodrug of paracetamol (acetaminophen) used for intravenous administration. It results from the combination of paracetamol and diethylglycine. It caused contact (hand and airborne) dermatitis in nurses, and acute systemic dermatitis (pompholyx and nummular dermatitis, generalized eczema, urticaria-like eruption) in nurses who had became sick and received intravenous propacetamol. Allergenic properties are due to the *N,N'*-diethylglycine moiety, and not to the paracetamol moiety. Propacetamol is now substituted by a solution of paracetamol in mannitol (Perfalgan®).

Suggested Reading
Barbaud A, Trechot P, Bertrand O, Schmutz JL (1995) Occupational allergy to propacetamol. Lancet 30:902
Berl V, Barbaud A, Lepoittevin JP (1998) Mechanism of allergic contact dermatitis from propacetamol: sensitization to activated *N,N*-diethylglycine. Contact Dermatitis 38:185–188
Le Coz C, Collet E, Dupouy M (1999) Conséquences d'une administration systémique de propacétamol (Pro-Dafalgan®) chez les infirmières sensibilisées au propacétamol. Ann Dermatol Venereol 126 [Suppl 2]: 32–33

342. Propargite

Omite®

CAS Registry Number [2312–35–8]

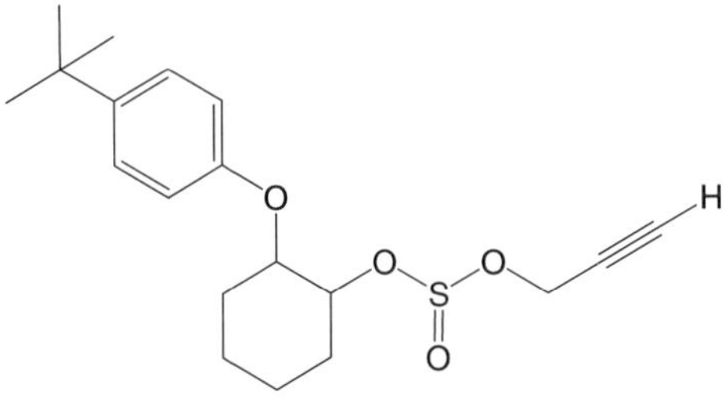

The pesticide omite principally acts as an irritant. Contact dermatitis was reported in 40 of 47 agricultural workers using Omite®.

Suggested Reading

Nishioka K, Kozuka T, Tashiro M (1970) Agricultural miticide (BPPS) dermatitis. Skin Res 12:15

O'Malley M, Rodriguez P, Maibach HI (1995) Pesticide patch testing: California nursery workers and controls. Contact Dermatitis 32:61–62

343. Propranolol

CAS Registry Number [525–66–6]

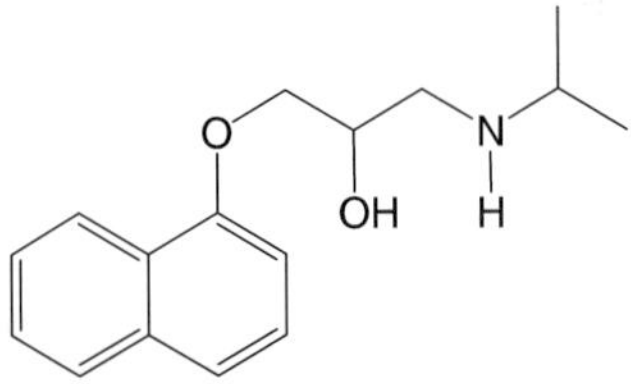

Propranolol is a beta-blocking agent that was responsible for the sensitization of workers in drug synthesis. In one case, epichlorhydrin was used for the production of drugs propranolol and oxprenolol. Cross-reactivity is expected between beta-blockers.

Suggested Reading

Pereira F, Dias M, Pacheco FA (1996) Occupational contact dermatitis from propranolol, hydralazine and bendroflumethiazide. Contact Dermatitis 35:303–304

Rebandel P, Rudzki E (1990) Dermatitis caused by epichlorhydrin, oxpren-olol hydrochloride and propranolol hydrochloride. Contact Dermatitis 23:199

344. Propyl Gallate

CAS Registry Number [121–79–9]

This gallate ester (E 311) is an antioxidant frequently used in the food, cosmetic, and pharmaceutical industries to prevent the oxidation of unsaturated fatty acids into rancid-smelling compounds. It causes cosmetic dermatitis mainly from lipsticks and induced contact dermatitis in a baker, and in a female confectioner, primarily sensitized by her night cream, who fried doughnuts – the margarine probably containing gallates.

Suggested Reading

Bojs G, Niklasson B, Svensson A (1987) Allergic contact dermatitis to propyl gallate. Contact Dermatitis 17:294–298

Marston S (1992) Propyl gallate on liposomes. Contact Dermatitis 27:74–76

Serra-Baldrich E, Puig LL, Gimenez Arnau A, Camarasa JG (1995) Lipstick allergic contact dermatitis from gallates. Contact Dermatitis 32:359–360

345. Propylene Glycol

1,2-Propanediol

CAS Registry Number [57–55–6]

Propylene glycol is used as a solvent, a vehicle for topical medicaments such as corticosteroids or aciclovir, an emulsifier and humectant in food and cosmetics, and as antifreeze in breweries, in the manufactures of resins. It was present as an occupational sensitizer in the color film developer Flexicolor®. Patch tests in aqua are sometimes irritant.

Suggested Reading

Claverie F, Giordano-Labadie F, Bazex J (1997) Eczéma de contact au propylène glycol. Ann Dermatol Venereol 124:315–317

Connoly M, Buckley DA (2004) Contact dermatitis from propylene glycol in ECG electrodes, complicated by medicament allergy. Contact Dermatitis 50:42

Scheman AJ, Katta R (1997) Photographic allergens: an update. Contact Dermatitis 37:130

346. Propylene Oxide

CAS Registry Number [75–56–9]

Propylene oxide is an allergic and irritant agent, used as a solvent and raw material in the chemical industry, as the starting material and intermediate for a broad spectrum of polymers. It can be used as a dehydrating agent for the preparation of slides in electron microscopy. Occupational dermatitis was also reported following the use of a skin disinfectant swab.

Suggested Reading

Steinkraus V, Hausen BM (1994) Contact allergy to propylene oxide. Contact Dermatitis 31:120

Van Ketel WG (1979) Contact dermatitis from propylene oxide. Contact Dermatitis 5:191–192

347. Pseudoephedrine

CAS Registry Number [90–82–4]

Pseudoephedrine Hydrochloride

CAS Registry Number [345–78–8]

Pseudoephedrine Sulfate

CAS Registry Number [7460–12–0]

This sympathomimetic α-adrenergic agonist is found in plants of the genus *Ephedra* (Ephedraceae) and is systemically used as a nasal decongestant. It can induce drug skin reactions such as acute generalized exanthematic pustulosis or generalized eczema.

Suggested Reading

Assier-Bonnet H, Viguier M, Dubertret L, Revuz J, Roujeau JC (2002) Severe adverse drug reactions due to pseudoephedrine from over-the-counter medications. Contact Dermatitis 47:165–182

Padial MA, Alvarez-Ferreira J, Tapia B, Blanco R, Manas C, Blanca M, Bellon T (2004) Acute generalized exanthematous pustulosis associated with pseudoephedrine. Br J Dermatol 150:139–142

348. Pyrethroids

Cypermethrin(e)

CAS Registry Number [52315–07–8]

Permethrin(e)

CAS Registry Number [52645–53–1]

Deltamethrin(e)

CAS Registry Number [52918–63–5]

Bioalletrhin(e), Depalethrin(e)

CAS Registry Number [584–79–2]

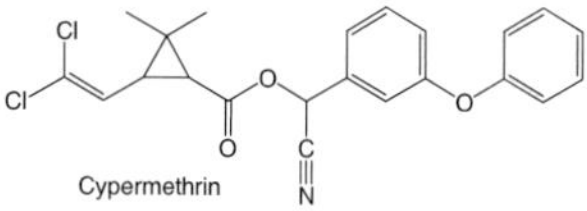

Cypermethrin

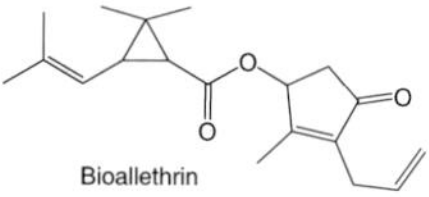

Bioallethrin

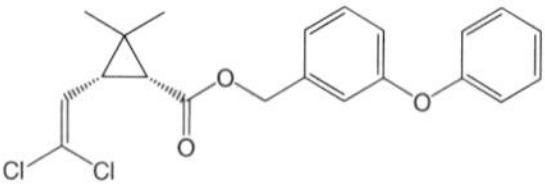

Permethrin

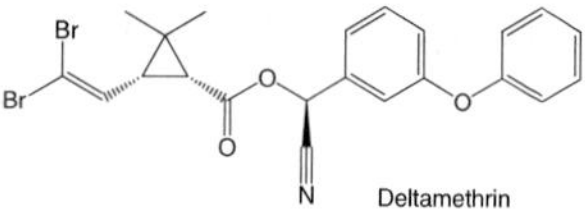

Deltamethrin

Pyrethroids, also called pyrethrinoids, are neurotoxic synthetic compounds used as insecticides, with irritant properties. Cyper-

methrin and fenvalerate have been reported as causing positive
allergic patch tests, but only fenvalerate was relevant in an agricultural worker.

Suggested Reading

Flannigan SA, Tucker SB, Key MM, Ross CE, Fairchild EJ 2nd, Grimes BA,
    Harrist RB (1985) Primary irritant contact dermatitis from synthetic
    pyrethroid insecticide exposure. Arch Toxicol 56:288–294
Lisi P (1992) Sensitization risk of pyrethroid insecticides. Contact Derma-
    titis 26:349–350

349. Pyrethrosin

CAS Registry Number [28272–18–6]

Pyrethrosin is an allergen of Asteraceae–Compositae such as
Chrysanthemum cinerariifolium Vis.

Suggested Reading

Mitchell JC, Dupuis G, Towers GHN (1972) Allergic contact dermatitis
    from pyrethrum (*Chrysanthemum* spp.). The roles of pyrethrosin, a
    sesquiterpene lactone, and of pyrethrin II. Br J Dermatol 86:568–573
Paulsen E, Andersen KE, Hausen BM (1993) Compositae dermatitis in a
    Danish dermatology department in one year (I). Results of routine
    patch testing with the sesquiterpene lactone mix supplemented with
    aimed patch testing with extracts and sesquiterpene lactones of Com-
    positae plants. Contact Dermatitis 29:6–10

350. Pyridine

CAS Registry Number [110–86–1]

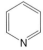

Pyridine (unsubstituted pyridine) and its derivative (substituted pyridines) are widely used in chemistry. Pyridine is a solvent used for many organic compounds and anhydrous metallic salt chemicals. Contained in Karl Fischer reagent, it induced contact dermatitis in a laboratory technician. No cross-sensitivity is observed between those different substances.

Suggested Reading

Knegt-Junk C, Geursen-Reitsma L, van Joost T (1993) Allergic contact dermatitis from pyridine in Karl Fischer reagent. Contact Dermatitis 28 : 252

351. Pyrithione

Pyrithione, Omadine

CAS Registry Number [1121–30–8]

Sodium Pyrithione, Sodium Omadine

CAS Registry Numbers [1121–30–8], [15922–78–8]

Zinc Pyrithione, Zinc Omadine

CAS Registry Number [13463–41–7] and more than 20 others

The sodium salt of N-hydroxy-2-pyridinethiones has germicidal activity against yeasts and fungi. Sodium omadine is a 40% aqueous solution of sodium pyrithione. It is used in the metallurgical industry as a component of water-based metalworking fluids, of aceto-polyvinyl lattices, water-based printer's ink, a lubricant for synthetic fibers and anti-dandruff shampoos.

Zinc pyrithione is widely used in anti-dandruff shampoos and is a classic allergen. Concomitant reactions are expected to both zinc and sodium pyrithione.

Suggested Reading

Le Coz CJ (2001) Allergic contact dermatitis from sodium pyrithione in metalworking fluid. Contact Dermatitis 45:58–59

Tosti A, Piraccini B, Brasile GP (1990) Occupational contact dermatitis due to sodium pyrithione. Contact Dermatitis 22:118–119

352. Pyrogallol

1,2,3-Benzenetriol, CI 76515, Pyrogallic Acid

CAS Registry Number [87–66–1]

Pyrogallol belongs to the phenols group. It is an old photograph developer and a low sensitizer in hair dyes.

Suggested Reading

Frosch PJ, Burrows D, Camarasa JG, Dooms-Goossens A, Ducombs G, Lahti A, Menné T, Rycroft RJG, Shaw S, White IR, Wilkinson JD (1993) Allergic reactions to a hairdresser's series: results from 9 European centres. Contact Dermatitis 28:180–183

Guerra L, Tosti A, Bardazzi F, Pigatto P, Lisi P, Santucci B, Valsecchi R, Schena D, Angelini G, Sertoli A, Ayala F, Kokelj F (1992) Contact dermatitis in hairdressers: the Italian experience. Gruppo Italiano Ricerca Dermatiti da Contatto e Ambientali. Contact Dermatitis 26:101–107

353. PVP

Polyvinylpyrrolidone, Polyvidone, Povidone, 2-Pyrrolidinone, 1-Ethenyl-, Homopolymer

CAS Registry Number [9003–39–8]

Polyvinylpyrrolidone is widely used as is in cosmetics such as hair care products, and in medical products. It acts as iodophor in iodine-polyvinylpyrrolidone. PVP is an irritant, and has been claimed as the allergen in some cases of dermatitis from iodine-polyvinylpyrrolidone (although iodine is more likely the hapten). It may cause type I contact urticaria or anaphylaxis.

Suggested Reading

Adachi A, Fukunaga A, Hayashi K, Kunisada M, Horikawa T (2003) Anaphylaxis to polyvinylpyrrolidone after vaginal application of povidone-iodine. Contact Dermatitis 48:133–136

Ronnau AC, Wulferink M, Gleichmann E, Unver E, Ruzicka T, Krutmann J, Grewe M (2000) Anaphylaxis to polyvinylpyrrolidone in an analgesic preparation. Br J Dermatol 143:1055–1058

354. PVP/Eicosene Copolymer

Polyvinylpyrrolidone/Eicosene Copolymer

CAS Registry Numbers [28211–18–9], [77035–98–4]

PVP/eicosene copolymer is the polymer of vinylpyrrolidone and of 1-eicosene, and one of the 11 PVP copolymers recorded in the International Nomenclature of Cosmetics Ingredients inventory system. This substance is utilized in cosmetics, in sunscreens to enhance their water resistance, and is an inert ingredient in pesticides. Contact sensitization to a close compound VP/eicosene copolymer was also reported.

Suggested Reading

Gallo R, dal Sacco D, Ghigliotti G (2004) Allergic contact dermatitis from VP/eisosene copolymer (Ganex® V-220) in an emollient cream. Contact Dermatitis 50:261

Le Coz CJ, Lefebvre C, Ludmann F, Grosshans E (2000) Polyvinylpyrrolidone (PVP)/eicosene copolymer: an emerging cosmetic allergen. Contact Dermatitis 43:61–62

355. PVP/Hexadecene Copolymer

CAS Registry Number
[32440–50–9]

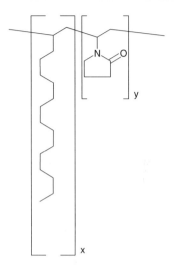

PVP/hexadecene copolymer, another PVP copolymer used for identical applications as PVP/eicosene copolymer, has been rarely implicated in contact dermatitis.

Suggested Reading

De Groot AC, Bruynzeel DP, Bos JD, van der Meeren HL, van Joost T, Jagtman BA, Weyland JW (1988) The allergens in cosmetics. Arch Dermatol 124 : 1525–1529

Scheman A, Cummins R (1998) Contact allergy to PVP/hexadecene copolymer. Contact Dermatitis 39 : 201

356. Quaternium-15

N-(3-Chloroallyl)Hexaminium Chloride, Hexamethylenetetramine Chloroallyl Chloride, Dowicil 200

CAS Registry Numbers [4080–31–3], [103638–29–5], [60789–82–4]

Quaternium-15 is a quaternary ammonium compound, used as a broad-spectrum formaldehyde-releasing bactericide agent. It is contained as a preservative in cosmetics, toiletries, and aqueous products. Allergy is mainly due to formaldehyde and not to Quaternium-15 itself. Occupational case reports concerned hairdressers, a beautician, an engineer working on the maintenance of machinery in a chicken processing plant, and an employee carrying out photocopying tasks.

Suggested Reading

Finch TM, Prais L, Foulds IS (2001) Occupational allergic contact dermatitis from quaternium-15 in an electroencephalography skin preparation gel. Contact Dermatitis 44:44–45

Marren P, de Berker D, Dawber RP, Powell S (1991) Occupational contact dermatitis due to quaternium 15 presenting as nail dystrophy. Contact Dermatitis 25:253–255

O'Reilly FM, Murphy GM (1996) Occupational contact dermatitis in a beautician. Contact Dermatitis 35:47–48

Tosti A, Piraccini BM, Bardazzi F (1990) Occupational contact dermatitis due to quaternium 15. Contact Dermatitis 23:41–42

Zina AM, Fanan E, Bundino S (2000) Allergic contact dermatitis from formaldehyde and quaternium-15 in photocopier toner. Contact Dermatitis 43:241–242

357. Quaternium-22

CAS Registry Numbers [51812–80–7], [82970–95–4]

This quaternary ammonium compound, used as a film former and conditioning agent, was reported as a co-sensitizer in eyelid dermatitis due to shellac-based mascara.

Suggested Reading

Le Coz CJ, Leclere JM, Arnoult E, Raison-Peyron N, Pons-Guiraud A, Vigan M, Members of Revidal-GERDA (2002) Allergic contact dermatitis from shellac in mascara. Contact Dermatitis 46:149–152

Scheman AJ (1998) Contact allergy to quaternium-22 and shellac in mascara. Contact Dermatitis 38:342–343

358. Ranitidine

CAS Registry Number [66357–35–5]

Ranitidine Hydrochloride

CAS Registry Number [66357–59–3]

Ranitidine, an H2-receptor antagonist, can cause contact dermatitis within the pharmaceutical industry and in healthcare workers, or may induce systemic drug reactions in patients.

Suggested Reading

Martinez MB, Salvador JF, Aguilera GV, Mas IB, Ramirez JC (2003) Acute generalized exanthematous pustulosis induced by ranitidine hydrochloride. Contact Dermatitis 49:47

Romaguerra C, Grimalt F, Vilaplana J (1988) Epidemic of occupational contact dermatitis from ranitidine. Contact Dermatitis 18:177–178

359. Resorcinol

1,3-Benzendiol, CI 76505

CAS Registry Number [108–46–3]

Resorcinol is used in hairdressing as a modifier (or a coupler) of the PPD group of dyes. It is the least frequent sensitizer in hairdressers. It is also used in resins, in skin treatment mixtures, and for tanning. Severe cases of dermatitis due to resorcinol contained in wart preparations have been reported.

Suggested Reading

Barbaud A, Modiano P, Cocciale M, Reichert S, Schmutz JL (1996) The topical application of resorcinol can provoke a systemic allergic reaction. Br J Dermatol 135:1014–1015

Frosch PJ, Burrows D, Camarasa JG, Dooms-Goossens A, Ducombs G,
Lahti A, Menné T, Rycroft RJG, Shaw S, White IR, Wilkinson JD (1993)
Allergic reactions to a hairdresser's series: results from 9 European
centres. Contact Dermatitis 28:180–183

Tarvainen K (1995) Analysis of patients with allergic patch test reactions
to a plastics and glue series. Contact Dermatitis 32:346–351

Vilaplana J, Romaguera C, Grimalt F (1991) Contact dermatitis from resorcinol in a hair dye. Contact Dermatitis 24:151–152

360. Silane

Monosilane

CAS Registry Number [7803–62–5] SiH_4

Various silane derivatives are used as bonding agents between
glass and the resin used as a coating agent of glass filaments.
Organosilanes have been implicated as sensitizers in workers at a
glass filament manufactory.

Suggested Reading
Heino T, Haapa K, Manelius F (1996) Contact sensitization to organos-
ilane solution in glass filament production. Contact Dermatitis 34:294

361. Sodium Bisulfite

Sodium Acid Sulfite, E222

CAS Registry Number [7631–90–5]

Sodium bisulfite is mainly used as an antioxidant in pharmaceutical products, as a disinfectant or bleach, and in the dye industry.
The bisulfite of commerce consists chiefly of metabisulfite, and
possesses the same properties as the true bisulfite. So, the allergen
to be tested in products containing disulfite is the corresponding
metabisulfite.

Suggested Reading
Budavari S, O'Neil MJ, Smith A, Heckelman PE, Kinneary JF (eds) (1996)
The Merck Index, 12th edn. Merck, Whitehouse Station, N.J., USA

362. Sodium lauryl sulfate

SLS, Sodium Dodecyl Sulfate

CAS Registry Number [151–21–3]

This anionic detergent is widely used in cosmetics and in industry. As a skin irritant agent, SLS can be used in several dermatological applications. It is also a good indicator of excited skin during patch testing.

Suggested Reading
Geier J, Uter W, Pirker C, Frosch PJ (2003) Patch testing with the irritant sodium lauryl sulfate (SLS) is useful in interpreting weak reactions to contact allergens as allergic or irritant. Contact Dermatitis 48:99–107

363. Sodium Metabisulfite

Sodium Pyrosulfite, Disodium Disulfite, E223

CAS Registry Number [7681–57–4]

This agent is frequently used as a preservative in pharmaceutical products, in the bread-making industry as an antioxidant, and it can induce contact dermatitis. It can be used as a reducing agent in photography and caused dermatitis in a photographic technician, probably acting as an aggravating irritative factor. Sodium metabisulfite contains a certain amount of sodium sulfite and sodium sulfate.

Suggested Reading
Acciai MC, Brusi C, Francalanci Giorgini S, Sertoli A (1993) Allergic contact dermatitis in caterers. Contact Dermatitis 28:48

Jacobs MC, Rycroft RJG (1995) Contact dermatitis and asthma from sodium metabisulfite in a photographic technician. Contact Dermatitis 33: 65–66

Riemersma WA, Schuttelaar ML, Coenraads PJ (2004) Type IV hypersensitivity to sodium metabisulfite in local anaesthetic. Contact Dermatitis 51:148

Vena GA, Foti C, Angelini G (1994) Sulfite contact allergy. Contact Dermatitis 31:172–175

364. Sodium Methyldithiocarbamate

Metham-Na, Carbathion, Sodium-*N*-Methyldithiocarbamate

CAS Registry Number [137–42–8]

Metham-Na is a fungicide nematocide of the dithiocarbamate group. Sensitization occurs among agricultural workers.

Suggested Reading

Koch P (1996) Occupational allergic contact dermatitis and airborne contact dermatitis from 5 fungicides in a vineyard worker. Cross-reactions between fungicides of the dithiocarbamate group? Contact Dermatitis 34:324–329

Pambor M, Bloch Y (1985) Dimethoat und Dithiocarmabat als berufliche Kontaktallergene bei einer Agrotechnikerin. Dermat Monatsschr 171: 401–405

Schubert H (1978) Contact dermatitis to sodium-*N*-methyldithiocarbamate. Contact Dermatitis 4:370–371

Wolf F, Jung HD (1970) Akute Kontaktdermatitiden nach Umgang mit Nematin. Z Ges Hyg 16:423–426

365. Sodium Sulfite

E225

CAS Registry Number [7757–83–7]]

Sodium sulfite is mainly used in photographic developers, for fixing prints, bleaching textile fibers, as a reducer in manufacturing dyes, as a remover of Cl in bleached textiles and paper, and as a preservative in the food industry for meat, egg yolks, and so on.

Suggested Reading

Budavari S, O'Neil MJ, Smith A, Heckelman PE, Kinneary JF (eds) (1996) The Merck Index, 12th edn. Merck, Whitehouse Station, N.J., USA

Vena GA, Foti C, Angelini G (1994) Sulfite contact allergy. Contact Dermatitis 31:172–175

366. Solvent Red 23

Sudan III, CI 26100, D and C Red No. 17

CAS Registry Number [85–86–9]

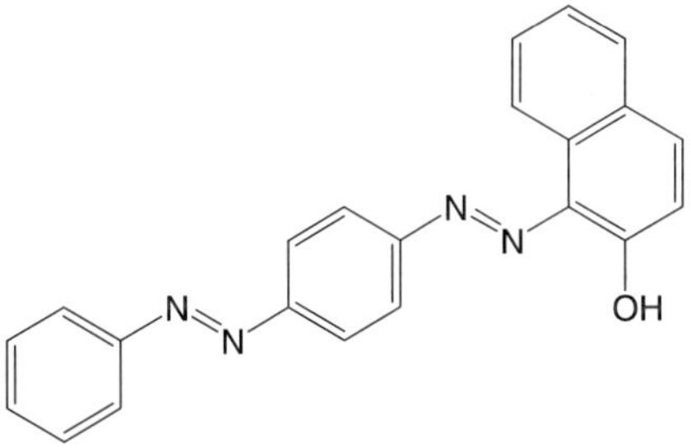

Solvent Red 23 is an oil-soluble red azo-dye used in cosmetic products in Japan. Cases were reported in hairdressers, who also reacted to PPD (the molecule is likely to be hydrolyzed into PPD) and to *p*-aminoazobenzene. One case of contact dermatitis was reported in the metal industry.

Suggested Reading

Fregert S (1967) Allergic contact dermatitis due to fumes from burning alcohol containing an azo-dye. Contact Dermatitis Newslett 1:11

Matsunaga K, Hayakawa R, Yoshimura K, Okada J (1990) Patch-test-positive reactions to Solvent Red 23 in hairdressers. Contact Dermatitis 23:266

367. Sorbitan Sesquioleate

Sorbitan 9-Octadecenoate (2:3), Arlacel 83, Anhydrohexitol Sesquioleate

CAS Registry Number [8007–43–0], [37318–79–9]

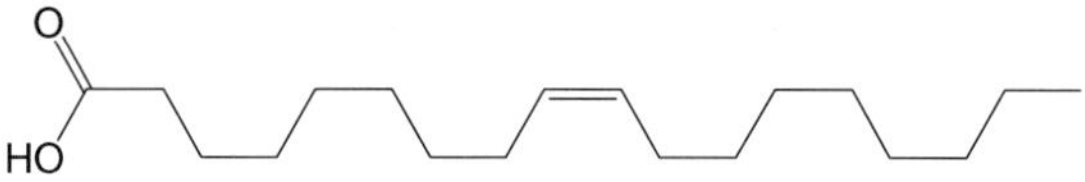

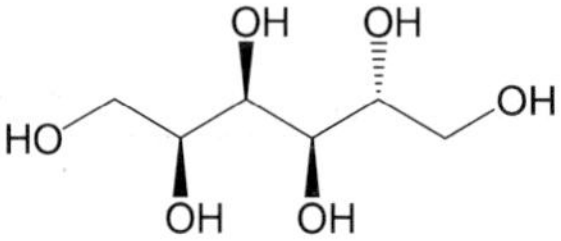

Sorbitan sesquioleate is a mixture of mono and diesters of oleic acid and extol anhydrides derived from sorbitol. It is used as a surfactant and an emulsifier in cosmetics. It acts sometimes as a contact allergen, particularly in leg ulcer patients. It is also responsible for false-positive patch test reactions to haptens, with which some allergen providers emulgated, such as parabens mix, fragrance mix, Amerchol L101, and ethylene-urea/melamine formaldehyde.

Suggested Reading

Orton DI, Shaw S (2001) Sorbitan sesquioleate as an allergen. Contact Dermatitis 44:190–191
Pasche-Koo F, Piletta PA, Hunziker N, Hauser C (1994) High sensitization rate to emulsifiers in patients with chronic leg ulcers. Contact Dermatitis 31:226–228

368. Spectinomycin

CAS Registry Number [1695–77–8]

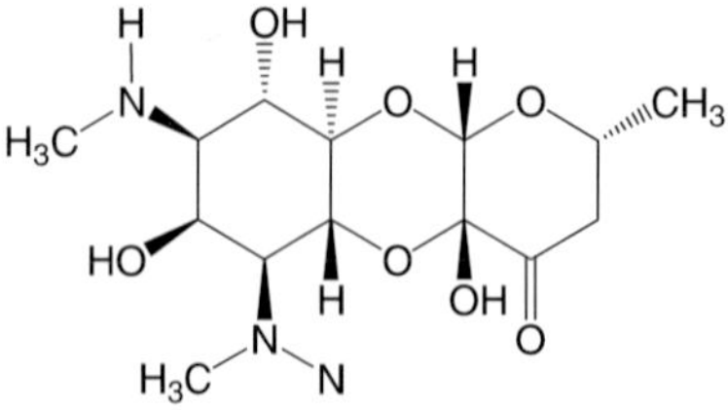

Spectinomycin is an aminocyclitol antibiotic. It is used in human medicine against *Neisseria gonorrhoeae* and in veterinary medicine, especially for poultry, pigs, and cattle. Cases of dermatitis have been reported in veterinary practice.

Suggested Reading

Dal Monte A, Laffi G, Mancini G (1994) Occupational contact dermatitis due to spectinomycin. Contact Dermatitis 31:204–205

Vilaplana J, Romaguera C, Grimalt F (1991) Contact dermatitis from lincomycin and spectinomycin in chicken vaccinators. Contact Dermatitis 24:225–226

369. Tetrabenzylthiuram Disulfide

TBzTD

CAS Registry Number
[10591–85–2]

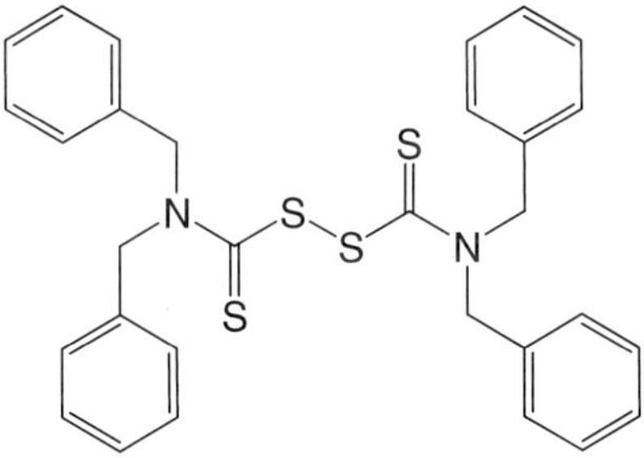

TBzTD is a rubber vulcanization accelerator.

Suggested Reading

Le Coz CJ (2004) Fiche d'éviction en cas d'hypersensibilité au thiuram mix. Ann Dermatol Venereol 131:1012–1014

370. Tetrabutylthiuram Disulfide

TBTD

CAS [1634–02–2]

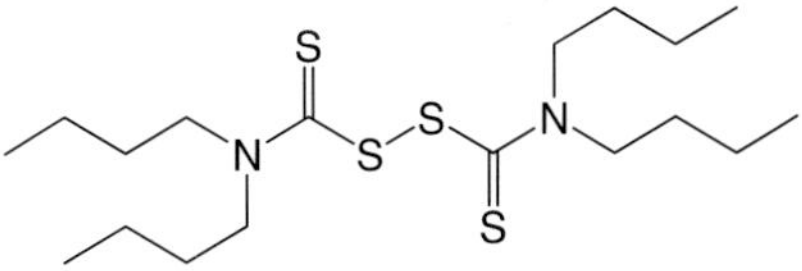

TBTD is a rubber vulcanization accelerator.

Suggested Reading

Le Coz CJ (2004) Fiche d'éviction en cas d'hypersensibilité au thiuram
    mix. Ann Dermatol Venereol 131:1012–1014

371. Tetrabutylthiuram Monosulfide

TBTM

CAS Registry Number
[97–74–5]

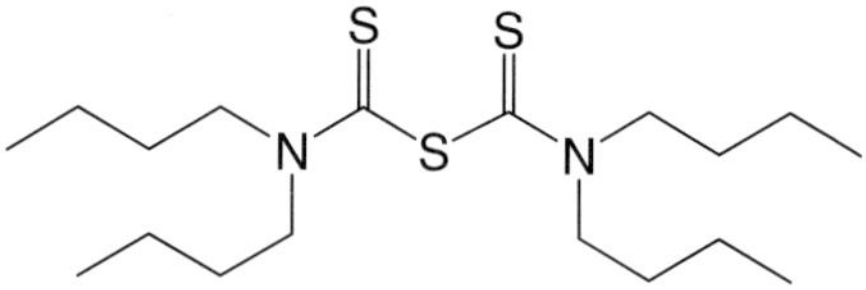

TBTM is a rubber vulcanization accelerator.

Suggested Reading

Le Coz CJ (2004) Fiche d'éviction en cas d'hypersensibilité au thiuram
    mix. Ann Dermatol Venereol 131:1012–1014

372. Tetrachloroacetophenone

CAS Registry Number
[39751–78–5]

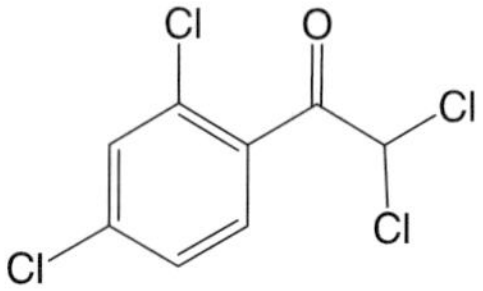

Tetrachloroacetophone was combined with triethyl phosphate to
form an organophosphate insecticide. It induced contact dermatitis in a process operator in an insecticide plant.

Suggested Reading

Van Joost T, Wiemer GR (1991) Contact dermatitis from tetrachloro-
    acetophenone (TCAP) in an insecticide plant. Contact Dermatitis 25:
    66–67

373. Tetraethylthiuram Disulfide

Disulfiram, TETD, Antabuse, Esperal®

CAS Registry Number
[97–77–8]

TETD is a rubber accelerator of the thiuram group, contained in "thiuram mix." It can cross-react with other thiurams, especially TMTD. TETD is used to aid those trying to break their dependence on alcohol. The disulfiram-alcohol reaction is not allergic but due to the accumulation of toxic levels of acetaldehyde. The implanted drug can, however, lead to local or generalized dermatitis, for example ingested disulfiram, mainly in previously rubber-sensitized patients. As an adjunctive treatment of alcoholism, it caused occupational contact dermatitis in a nurse.

Suggested Reading

Condé-Salazar L, Del-Rio E, Guimaraens D, Gonzalez Domingo A (1993) Type IV allergy to rubber additives: a 10-year study of 686 cases. J Am Acad Dermatol 29:176–180

Kiec-Swierczynska M, Krecisz B, Fabicka B (2000) Systemic contact dermatitis from implanted disulfiram. Contact Dermatitis 43(4):246–247

Le Coz CJ (2004) Fiche d'éviction en cas d'hypersensibilité au thiuram mix. Ann Dermatol Venereol 131:1012–1014

Mathelier-Fusade P, Leynadier F (1994) Occupational allergic contact reaction to disulfiram. Contact Dermatitis 31:121–122

Webb PK, Bibbs SC (1979) Disulfiram hypersensitivity and rubber contact dermatitis. JAMP 241:2061

374. Tetraethylthiuram Monosulfide

Sulfiram, TETM, Tetraethylthiodicarbonic Diamide

CAS Registry Number
[95–05–6]

This rubber vulcanization accelerator is also used as an ectoparasiticide against *Sarcoptes scabiei*, louses or in veterinary medicine.

Suggested Reading
Le Coz CJ (2004) Fiche d'éviction en cas d'hypersensibilité au thiuram mix. Ann Dermatol Venereol 131 : 1012–1014

375. Tetraisobutylthiuram Disulfide

TITD, Thioperoxydicarbonic Diamide, Tetrakis (2-Methylpropyl)

CAS Registry Number [137–26–8]

TITD is a rubber vulcanization accelerator.

Suggested Reading
Le Coz CJ (2004) Fiche d'éviction en cas d'hypersensibilité au thiuram mix. Ann Dermatol Venereol 131 : 1012–1014

376. Tetramethylthiuram Disulfide

Thiram, TMTD

CAS Registry Number [137–26–8]

This rubber chemical, accelerator of vulcanization, represents the most commonly positive allergen contained in "thiuram mix." The most frequent occupational categories are the metal industry, homemakers, health services and laboratories, the building industry, and shoemakers. It is also widely used as a fungicide, belonging to the dithiocarbamate group of carrots, bulbs, and woods, and as an insecticide. Thiram is the agricultural name for thiuram.

Suggested Reading

Condé-Salazar L, Guimaraens D, Villegas C, Romero A, Gonzalez MA (1995) Occupational allergic contact dermatitis in construction workers. Contact Dermatitis 35:226–230

Kiec-Swierczynska M (1995) Occupational sensitivity to rubber. Contact Dermatitis 32:171–172

Le Coz CJ (2004) Fiche d'éviction en cas d'hypersensibilité au thiuram mix. Ann Dermatol Venereol 131:1012–1014

Mancuso G, Reggiani M, Berdondini RM (1996) Occupational dermatitis in shoemakers. Contact Dermatitis 34:17–22

Sharma VK, Kaur S (1990) Contact sensitization by pesticides in farmers. Contact Dermatitis 23:77–80

377. Tetramethylthiuram Monosulfide

TMTM

CAS Registry Number [97–74–5]

This rubber accelerator is contained in "thiuram mix." The most frequent occupational categories are the metal industry, homemakers, health services and laboratories, and the building industry.

Suggested Reading

Condé-Salazar L, Del-Rio E, Guimaraens D, Gonzalez Domingo A (1993) Type IV allergy to rubber additives: a 10-year study of 686 cases. J Am Acad Dermatol 29:176–180

Condé-Salazar L, Guimaraens D, Villegas C, Romero A, Gonzalez MA (1995) Occupational allergic contact dermatitis in construction workers. Contact Dermatitis 35:226–230

Le Coz CJ (2004) Fiche d'éviction en cas d'hypersensibilité au thiuram mix. Ann Dermatol Venereol 131:1012–1014

Von Hintzenstern J, Heese A, Koch HU, Peters KP, Hornstein OP (1991) Frequency, spectrum and occupational relevance of type IV allergies to rubber chemicals. Contact Dermatitis 24:244–252

378. Tetrazepam

CAS Registry Number [10379–14–3]

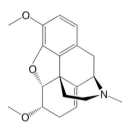

Tetrazepam is a benzodiazepine compound used systemically as a myorelaxant. It may induce skin rashes such as maculo-papular eruption, Stevens–Johnson syndrome or photosensitivity. Occupational sensitization can be observed in pharmaceutical plants. Sensitization generally does not concern other benzodiazepines (personal observations).

Suggested Reading

Barbaud A, Trechot P, Reichert-Penetrat S, Granel F, Schmutz JL (2001) The usefulness of patch testing on the previously most severely affected site in a cutaneous adverse drug reaction to tetrazepam. Contact Dermatitis 44:259–260

Choquet-Kastylevsky G, Testud F, Chalmet P, Lecuyer-Kudela S, Descotes J (2001) Occupational contact allergy to tetrazepam. Contact Dermatitis 44:372

379. Thebaine

CAS Registry Number [115–37–7]

The naturally occurring opiate alkaloid thebaine is present in concentrated poppy straw, and in small concentrations in codeine alkaloid. It is used in the manufacture of other opiate pharmaceuticals, such as buprenorphine and morphine, and caused contact dermatitis in a laboratory worker at an opiates manufacturing pharmaceutical company, also sensitive to codeine.

Suggested Reading

Waclawski ER, Aldridge R (1995) Occupational dermatitis from thebaine and codeine. Contact Dermatitis 33:51

380. Thiabendazole

CAS Registry Number [148–79–8]

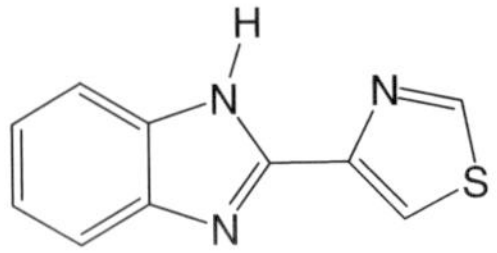

This fungicide and vermifuge agent is widely used in agriculture (for example, for citrus fruits), and in medical and veterinary practice as an anthelmintic drug.

Suggested Reading

Izu R, Aguirre A, Goicoechea A, Gardeazabal J, Diaz Perez JL (1993) Photoaggravated allergic contact dermatitis due to topical thiabendazole. Contact Dermatitis 28:243–244

Mancuso G, Staffa M, Errani A, Berdondini RM, Fabri P (1990) Occupational dermatitis in animal feed mill workers. Contact Dermatitis 22: 37–41

381. Thimerosal

Thiomersal, Thiomersalate, Merthiolate, Mercurothiolic Acid Sodium Salt

CAS Registry Number [54–64–8]

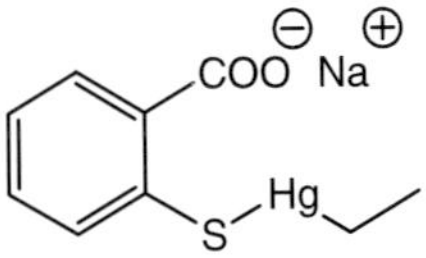

Thiomersal is an organic mercury salt prepared by reacting ethylmercuric chloride (or ethylmercuric hydroxide) with thiosalicylic acid. It is still used as a disinfectant and a preservative agent, but less commonly than previously, especially in contact lens fluids, eyedrops, and vaccines. The ethylmercuric moiety is the major allergenic determinant, sometimes associated with mercury sensitivity. Thiomersal is an indicator of photosensitivity to piroxicam, through its thiosalicylic moiety.

Suggested Reading

Arévalo A, Blancas R, Ancona A (1995) Occupational contact dermatitis from piroxicam. Am J Contact Dermat 6:113–114

De Groot AC, van Wijnen WG, van Wijnen-Vos M (1990) Occupational contact dermatitis of the eyelids, without ocular involvement, from thimerosal in contact lens fluid. Contact Dermatitis 23:195

Rudzki E, Rebandel P, Grzywa Z, Pomorski Z, Jakiminska B, Zawisza E (1982) Occupational dermatitis in veterinarians. Contact Dermatitis 8 :72–73

382. Thiourea

Thiocarbamide

CAS Registry Number [62–56–6]

Thiourea is used as a cleaner agent for silver and copper, and as an antioxidant in diazo copy paper. It can induce (photo-)contact dermatitis.

Suggested Reading

Dooms-Goossens A, Debusschère K, Morren M, Roelandts R, Coopman S (1988) Silver polish: another source of contact dermatitis reactions to thiourea. Contact Dermatitis 19:133–135

Geier J, Fuchs T (1993) Contact allergy due to 4-N,N-dimethylamino-benzene diazonium chloride and thiourea in diazo copy paper. Contact Dermatitis 28:304–305

Kanerva L, Estlander T, Jolanki R (1994) Occupational allergic contact dermatitis caused by thiourea compounds. Contact Dermatitis 31: 242–248

383. Thymoquinone

CAS Registry Number [490–91–5]

Thymoquinone is an allergen in different cedar species, Cupressaceae family, such as incense cedar (*Calocedrus decurrens* Florin) used for pencils, chests or toys, and western cedar (*Thuja plicata* Donn.) as used for hard realizations such as construction or boats.

Suggested Reading

Hausen BM (2000) Woods. In: Kanerva L, Elsner P, Wahlberg JE, Maibach HI (eds) Handbook of occupational dermatology. Springer, Berlin Heidelberg New York, pp 771–780

Lamminpää A, Estlander T, Jolanki R, Kanerva L (1996) Occupational allergic contact dermatitis caused by decorative plants. Contact Dermatitis 34:330–335

384. Timolol

CAS Registry Number [26839–75–8]

Timolol was implicated in allergic contact dermatitis due to beta-blocker agents in eyedrops.

Suggested Reading

Giordano-Labadie F, Lepoittevin JP, Calix I, Bazex J (1997) Allergie de contact aux â-bloqueurs des collyres: allergie croisée? Ann Dermatol Venereol 124:322–324

385. Tixocortol Pivalate

Tixocortol 21-Pivalate, Tixocortol 21-Trimethylacetate

CAS Registry Number [55560–96–8]

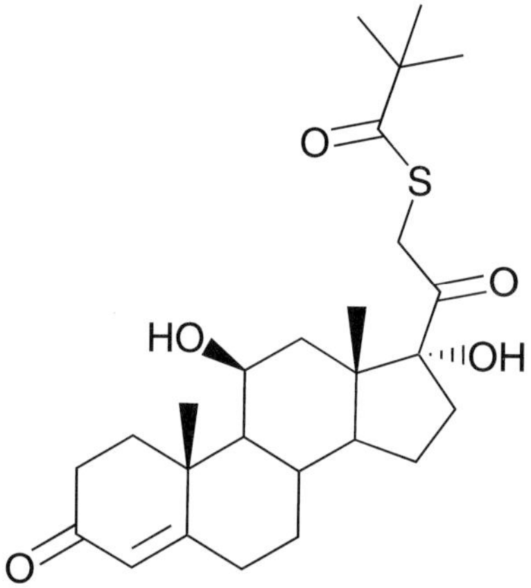

Tixocortol 21-pivalate is a 21-ester of tixocortol, widely used in topical treatments. It can induce severe allergic contact dermatitis. This corticosteroid is a marker of the allergenic A group that includes molecules without major substitution on the D cycle (no C_{16} methylation, no C_{17} side chain). A short-chain C_{21} ester is possible. Molecules are cloprednol, cortisone, fludrocortisone, fluorometholone, hydrocortisone, methylprednisolone, methylprednisone, prednisolone, prednisone, tixocortol, and their C_{21} esters (acetate, caproate or hexanoate, phosphate, pivalate or trimethylacetate, succinate or hemisuccinate, m-sulfobenzoate).

Suggested Reading

Le Coz CJ (2002) Fiche d'éviction en cas d'hypersensibilité au pivalate de tixocortol. Ann Dermatol Venereol 129:348–349

Lepoittevin JP, Drieghe J, Dooms-Goossens A (1995) Studies in patients with corticosteroid contact allergy. Understanding cross-reactivity among different steroids. Arch Dermatol 131:31–37

386. Tocopherol, Tocopheryl Acetate (DL-, D-)

Vitamin E

CAS Registry Number [1406–66–2,]

Vitamin E Acetate DL, Vitamin E Acetate D

CAS Registry Number [7695–91–2],
CAS Registry Number [58–95–7]

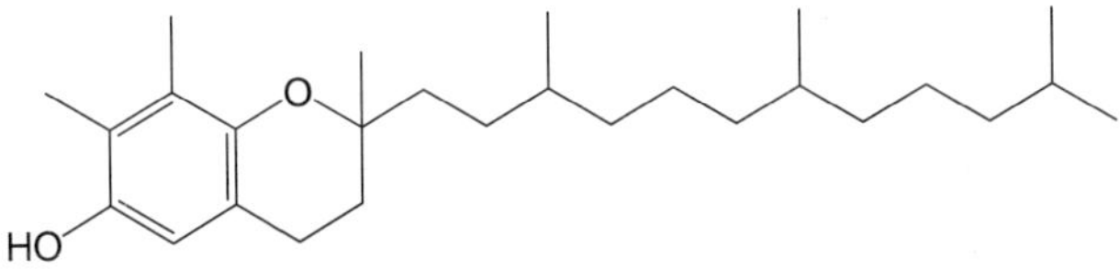

Tocopherol and tocopheryl acetate are used mainly as antioxidants. Tocopheryl acetate, an ester of tocopherol (vitamin E), can induce allergic contact dermatitis.

Suggested Reading

De Groot AC, Berretty PJ, van Ginkel CJ, den Hengst CW, van Ulsen J, Weyland JW (1991) Allergic contact dermatitis from tocopheryl acetate in cosmetic creams. Contact Dermatitis 25:302–304

Matsumura T, Nakada T, Iijima M (2004) Widespread contact dermatitis from tocopherol acetate. Contact Dermatitis 51:211–212

387. Toluene-2,5-Diamine

p-Toluylenediamine, *p*-Toluenediamine

CAS Registry Number
[95–70–5]

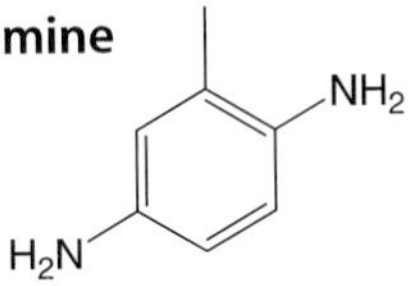

Toluene-2,5-diamine is a permanent hair dye involved in contact dermatitis in hairdressers and consumers. It does not cross-react with PPD, but co-sensitization is frequent.

Suggested Reading

Frosch PJ, Burrows D, Camarasa JG, Dooms-Goossens A, Ducombs G, Lahti A, Menné T, Rycroft RJG, Shaw S, White IR, Wilkinson JD (1993) Allergic reactions to a hairdresser's series: results from 9 European centres. Contact Dermatitis 28:180–183

Guerra L, Tosti A, Bardazzi F, Pigatto P, Lisi P, Santucci B, Valsecchi R, Schena D, Angelini G, Sertoli A, Ayala F, Kokelj F (1992) Contact dermatitis in hairdressers: the Italian experience. Gruppo Italiano Ricerca Dermatiti da Contatto e Ambientali. Contact Dermatitis 26:101–107

Le Coz CJ, Lefebvre C, Keller F, Grosshans E (2000) Allergic contact dermatitis caused by skin painting (pseudotattooing) with black henna, a mixture of henna and *p*-phenylenediamine and its derivatives. Arch Dermatol 136:1515–1517

388. Toluene Diisocyanate

Toluene Diisocyanate (Mixture)

CAS Registry Number [26471–62–5]

Toluene 2,4-Diisocyanate

CAS Registry Number [584–84–9]

Toluene 2,6-Diisocyanate

CAS Registry Number [91–08–7]

2,4-TDI   2,6-TDI

Toluene diisocyanate is a mixture of 2,4-TDI and 2,6-TDI. It is used in the manufacture of various polyurethane products: elastic and rigid foams, paints, lacquers, adhesives, binding agents, synthetics rubbers, and elastomeric fibers.

Suggested Reading

Estlander T, Keskinen H, Jolanki R, Kanerva L (1992) Occupational dermatitis from exposure to polyurethane chemicals. Contact Dermatitis 27: 161–165

Le Coz CJ, El Aboubi S, Ball C (1999) Active sensitization to toluene di-isocyanate. Contact Dermatitis 41:104–105

389. Tosyl Chloride

p-Toluene Sulfonyl Chloride, *p*-Toluene Sulfochloride

CAS Registry Number [98–59–9].

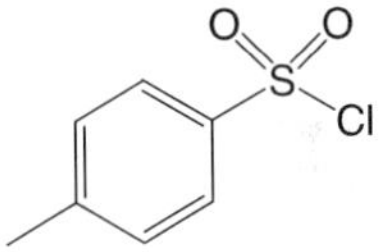

Tosyl chloride is used mainly in the preparation of chemical derivatives in the pharmaceutical, plastics, and organic chemical industries.

Suggested Reading

Watsky KL, Reynolds K, Berube D, Bayer FJ (1993) Occupational contact dermatitis from tosyl chloride in a chemist. Contact Dermatitis 29: 211–212

390. Triacetin

Glyceryl Triacetate

CAS Registry Number [102–76–1]

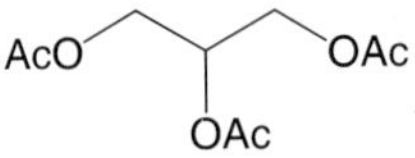

Triacetin is a component of cigarette filters, which induced a contact dermatitis in a worker at a cigarette manufactory.

Suggested Reading

Unna PJ, Schulz KH (1963) Allergisches Kontaktekzem durch Triacetin. Hautarzt 14: 423–425

391. Tributyltin Oxide

CAS Registry Number [56–35–9]

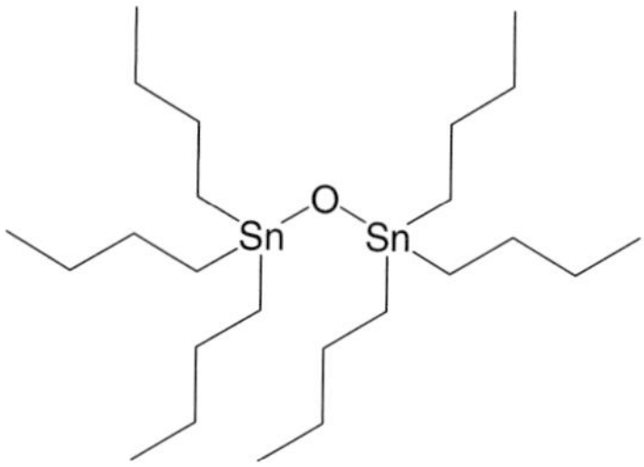

Tributyl tin oxide is used as an antifouling and biocide agent against fungi, algae, and bacteria, particularly in paints. Sometimes used in chemistry, tributyltin oxide is a strong irritant.

Suggested Reading

Goh CL (1985) Irritant dermatitis from tri-*N*-butyl tin oxide in paint. Contact Dermatitis 12 : 161–163

Grace CT, Ng SK, Cheong LL (1991) Recurrent irritant contact dermatitis due to tributyltin oxide on work clothes. Contact Dermatitis 25 : 250–251

392. Trichloroethane

1,1,1-Trichloroethane, Methylchloroform

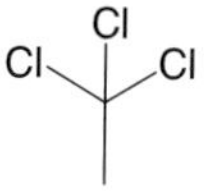

CAS Registry Numbers [71–55–6], [25323–89–1]

Trichloroethane is a solvent that has wide applications in industry, such as for cold type metal cleaning, and in cleaning plastic molds. It is mainly an irritant but can also provoke allergic contact dermatitis.

Suggested Reading

Mallon J, Tek Chu M, Maibach HI (2001) Occupational allergic contact dermatitis from methyl chloroform (1,1,1-trichloroethane)? Contact Dermatitis 45 : 107

393. Trichloroethylene

Trilene, Triclene, Trethylene

CAS Registry Number [79–01–6]

Trichloroethylene is a chlorinated hydrocarbon used as a detergent or solvent for metals, oils, resins, sulfur and as general degreasing agent. It can cause irritant contact dermatitis, generalized exanthema, Stevens–Johnson-like syndrome, pustular or bullous eruption, scleroderma, as well as neurological and hepatic disorders.

Suggested Reading

Goon AT, Lee LT, Tay YK, Yosipovitch G, Ng SK, Giam YC (2001) A case of trichloroethylene hypersensitivity syndrome. Arch Dermatol 137: 274–276

Puerschel WC, Odia SG, Rakoski J, Ring J (1996) Trichloroethylene and concomitant contact dermatitis in an art painter. Contact Dermatitis 34: 430–431

394. Triethanolamine

Trolamine

CAS Registry Number [102–71–6]

This emulsifying agent can be contained in many products such as cosmetics, topical medicines, metalworking cutting fluids, and color film developers. Traces may exist in other ethanolamines such as mono- and diethanolamine. Contact allergy seems to be rarer than previously thought.

Suggested Reading

Blum A, Lischka G (1997) Allergic contact dermatitis from mono-, di- and triethanolamine. Contact Dermatitis 36: 166

Le Coz CJ, Scrivener Y, Santinelli F, Heid E (1998) Sensibilisation de contact au cours des ulcères de jambe. Ann Dermatol Venereol 125: 694–699

Scheman AJ, Katta R (1997) Photographic allergens: an update. Contact Dermatitis 37: 130

395. Triethylenetetramine

CAS Registry Number [112–24–3]

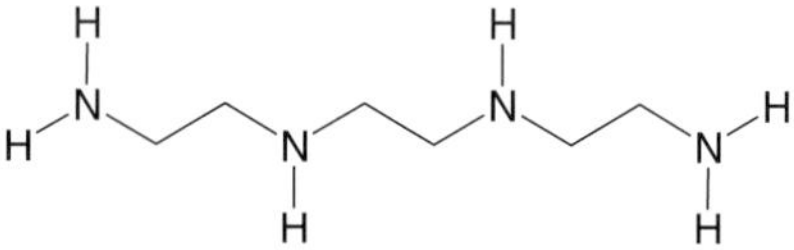

Triethylenetetramine is used as an amine hardener in epoxy resins of the bisphenol A type. Cross-sensitivity is possible with diethylenetriamine and diethylenediamine.

Suggested Reading

Jolanki R, Kanerva L, Estlander T, Tarvainen K, Keskinen H, Henriks-Eckerman ML (1990) Occupational dermatoses from epoxy resin compounds. Contact Dermatitis 23:172–183

396. Triforine

Saprol®,
1,4-bis(2,2,2-Trichloro-1-Formamidoethyl)Piperazine

CAS Registry Number [26644–46–2]

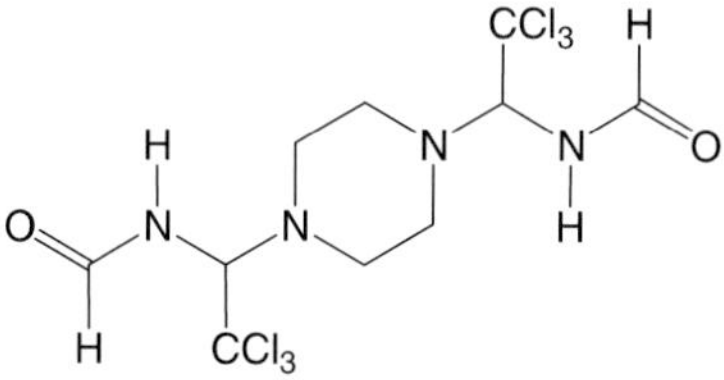

This pesticide is widely used in flower growing. Cross-reactions are expected to dichlorvos.

Suggested Reading

Ueda A, Aoyama K, Manda F, Ueda T, Kawahara Y (1994) Delayed-type allergenicity of triforine (Saprol®). Contact Dermatitis 31:140–145

397. Triglycidyl Isocyanurate

1,3,5-Triglycidyl-*s*-Triazinetrione

CAS Registry Number [2451–62–9]

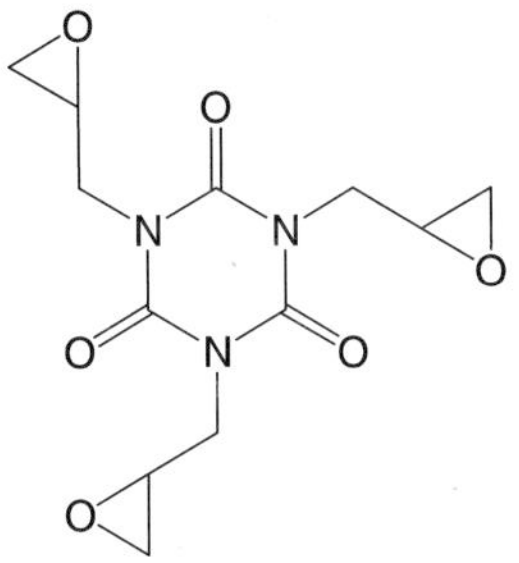

Triglycidyl isocyanurate is a triazine epoxy compound used as a resin hardener in polyester powder paints, in the plastics industry, resin molding systems, inks, and adhesives. Occupational contact dermatitis can occur in people producing this chemical, in those producing the powder coat paint, and in sprayers. Respiratory symptoms have been observed.

Suggested Reading

Erikstam U, Bruze M, Goossens A (2001) Degradation of triglycidyl isocyanurate as a cause of false-negative patch test reaction. Contact Dermatitis 44:13–17

Foulds IS, Koh D (1992) Allergic contact dermatitis from resin hardeners during the manufacture of thermosetting coating paints. Contact Dermatitis 26:87–90

McFadden JP, Rycroft RJG (1993) Occupational contact dermatitis from triglycidyl isocyanurate in a powder paint sprayer. Contact Dermatitis 28:251

Munro CS, Lawrence CM (1992) Occupational contact dermatitis from triglycidyl isocyanurate in a powder paint factory. Contact Dermatitis 26:59

398. *N*-[3-(Trimethoxysilyl)Propyl]-*N*'-(Vinylbenzyl) Ethylenediamine Monohydrochloride

1,2-Ethanediamine, *N*-[(Ethenylphenyl)Methyl]-*N*'-[3-(Trimethoxysilyl)Propyl]-, Monohydrochloride

HCl

This amine-functional methoxysilane silane compound, referenced as vinylbenzylaminoethyl aminopropyltrimethoxysilane, was implicated in the production of glass filaments.

Suggested Reading

Heino T, Haapa K, Manelius F (1996) Contact sensitization to organo-silane solution in glass filament production. Contact Dermatitis 34:294

Toffoletto F, Cortona G, Feltrin G, Baj A, Goggi E, Cecchetti R (1994) Occupational contact dermatitis from amine-functional methoxysilane in continuous-glass-filament production. Contact Dermatitis 31:320–321

399. *N*-(3-Trimethoxysilylpropyl)-Ethylenediamine

Z 6020

CAS Registry Number
[1760–24–3]

This amine-functional methoxysilane, referenced as aminoethyl aminopropyltrimethoxysilane, was implicated in the production of glass filaments.

Suggested Reading

Heino T, Haapa K, Manelius F (1996) Contact sensitization to organo-silane solution in glass filament production. Contact Dermatitis 34:294

400. 2,4,6-Trimethylol Phenol

CAS Registry Number [2937–61–3]

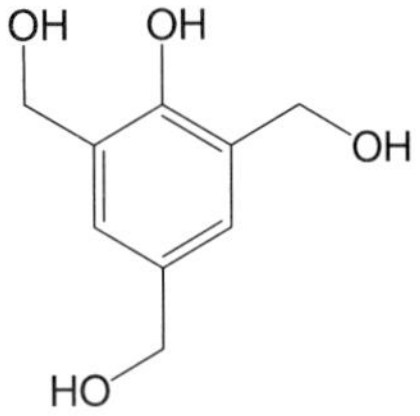

Trimethylolphenol is an allergen in resins based on phenol and formaldehyde. Cross-reactivity is possible with other phenol-derivative molecules.

Suggested Reading

Bruze M, Zimerson E (1997) Cross-reaction patterns in patients with contact allergy to simple methylol phenols. Contact Dermatitis 37 : 82–86

Bruze M, Fregert S, Zimerson E (1985) Contact allergy to phenol-formaldehyde resins. Contact Dermatitis 12 : 81–86

401. Trimethylthiourea

CAS Registry Number [2489–77–2]

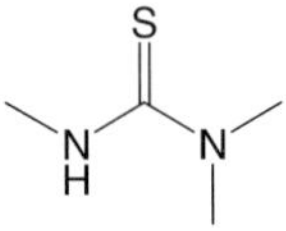

Trimethylthiourea is a thiourea derivative used for polychloroprene (neoprene) rubber vulcanization, for example. Patients sensitized to ethylbutyl thiourea can also react to trimethylthiourea.

Suggested Reading

Kanerva L, Estlander T, Jolanki R (1994) Occupational allergic contact dermatitis caused by thiourea compounds. Contact Dermatitis 31 : 242–248

402. Tulipalin A and Tulipalin B

α-Methylene-γ-Butyrolactone
and β-Hydroxy-α-Methylene-γ-Butyrolactone

CAS Registry Number [547–65–9]
and CAS Registry Number [38965–80–9]

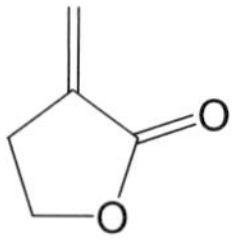

Tulipalin A 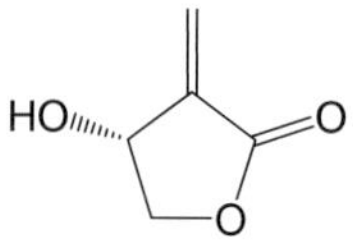   Tulipalin B

Tulipalin A is the unsubstituted α-methylene-γ-butyrolactone contained in the sap of damaged tulips (Liliaceae family) and Alstroemeria (Alstroemeriaceae family). Tulipalin B, due to hydrolysis of tuliposide B, seems to have a weak sensitizing capacity.

Suggested Reading

Bruynzeel DP (1997) Bulb dermatitis. Dermatological problems in the flower bulb industries. Contact Dermatitis 37:70–77

Gette MT, Marks JE (1990) Tulip fingers. Arch Dermatol 126:203–205

403. Tuliposide A

CAS Registry Number [19870–30–5]

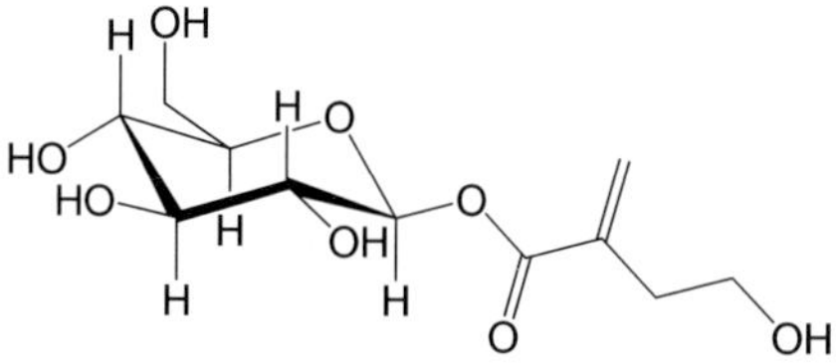

Tuliposide A is a glucoside prohapten contained in tulip bulbs and in Alstroemeria (*Tulipa* spp.; *Alstroemeria* spp.; *Lilium* spp.). It is rapidly hydrolyzed to tulipalin A and represents a common occupational problem among workers in the European tulip industry. Tuliposide can be present as 1-tuliposide A, but is more frequently identified as 6-tuliposide A.

Suggested Reading

Christensen LP, Kristiansen K (1995) A simple HPLC method for the isolation and quantification of the allergens tuliposide A and tulipalin A in
Alstroemeria. Contact Dermatitis 32:199–203

Gette MT, Marks JE (1990) Tulip fingers. Arch Dermatol 126:203–205

Lamminpää A, Estlander T, Jolanki R, Kanerva L (1996) Occupational allergic contact dermatitis caused by decorative plants. Contact Dermatitis
34:330–335

404. Tylosin

CAS Registry Number [1401-69-0]

Tylosin is a macrolid antibiotic used in veterinary medicine.
Occupational exposure concerns farmers, breeders, animal feed
workers, and veterinarians.

Suggested Reading

Barbera E, de la Cuadra J (1989) Occupational airborne allergic contact
dermatitis from tylosin. Contact Dermatitis 20:308–309

Carafini S, Assalve D, Stingeni L, Lisi P (1994) Tylosin, an airborne contact
allergen in veterinarians. Contact Dermatitis 31:327–328

Guerra L, Venturo N, Tardio M, Tosti A (1991) Airborne contact dermatitis
from animal feed antibiotics. Contact Dermatitis 25:333–334

Tuomi ML, Räsänen L (1995) Contact allergy to tylosin and cobalt in a pig-
farmer. Contact Dermatitis 33:285

405. Urushil

CAS Registry Number [492–89–7], [53237–59–5]

Urushiol is a generic name that indicates a mixture of several close alkylcatechols contained in the sap of the Anacardiaceae family such as *Toxicodendron radicans* Kuntze (poison ivy) or *Anacardium occidentale* L. (cashew nut tree). The R-side chain generally includes 13, 15 or 17 carbons. A urushiol with a C_{15} side chain is named pentadecylcatechol (a term sometimes employed in medical literature for poison ivy urushiol), and a urushiol with a C_{17} side chain is a heptadecylcatechol (mostly encountered in poison oak urushiol).

Suggested Reading

Epstein WL (1994) Occupational poison ivy and oak dermatitis. Dermatol Clin 12:511–516

Kawai K, Nakagawa M, Kawai K, Konishi K, Liew FM, Yasuno H, Shimode Y, Shimode Y (1991) Hyposensitization to urushiol among Japanese lacquer craftsmen. Contact Dermatitis 24:146–147

Kullavanijaya P, Ophaswongse S (1997) A study of dermatitis in the lacquerware industry. Contact Dermatitis 36:244–246

406. Usnic Acid (D-Usnic Acid, L-Usnic Acid)

CAS Registry Number [125–46–2]
(CAS Registry Number [7562–61–0],
CAS Registry Number [6159–66–6])

Usnic acid is a component of lichens, also used as a topical antibiotic. Allergic contact dermatitis from lichens occurs mainly occupationally in forestry and horticultural workers, and in lichen pickers.

Suggested Reading

Aalto-Korte K, Lauerma A, Alanko K (2005) Occupational allergic contact dermatitis from lichens in present-day Finland. Contact Dermatitis 52 : 36–38

Hahn M, Lischka G, Pfeifle J, Wirth V (1995) A case of contact dermatitis from lichens in southern Germany. Contact Dermatitis 32 : 55–56

407. Vinylpyridine

2-Vinylpyridine

CAS Registry Number [100–69–6]

4-Vinylpyridine

CAS Registry Number [100–43–6]

2-VP   4-VP

4-Vinyl pyridine was used as a monomer in polymer chemistry and induced nonimmunological contact urticaria, and allergic contact dermatitis. No cross-reactivity is observed between pyridine derivatives.

Suggested Reading

Bergendorff O, Wallengren J (1999) 4-Vinylpyridine-induced dermatitis in a laboratory worker. Contact Dermatitis 40 : 280–281

Foussereau J, Lantz JP, Grosshans E (1972) Allergic eczema from vinyl-4-pyridine. Contact Dermatitis Newslett 11 : 261

Sasseville D, Balbul A, Kwong P, Yu K (1996) Contact sensitization to pyridine derivatives. Contact Dermatitis 35 : 101–102

408. Virginiamycin

CAS Registry Number [11006–76–1]

Virginiamycin S1: Staphylomycin S

CAS Registry Number [23152–29–6]

Virginiamycin M1: Pristinamycin IIA, Mikamycin A, Ostreogrycin A,
Staphylomycin M1, Streptogramin A, Vernamycin A

CAS Registry Number [21411–53–0]

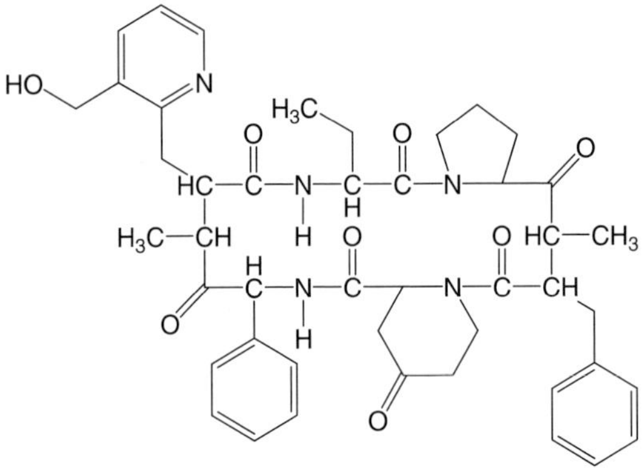

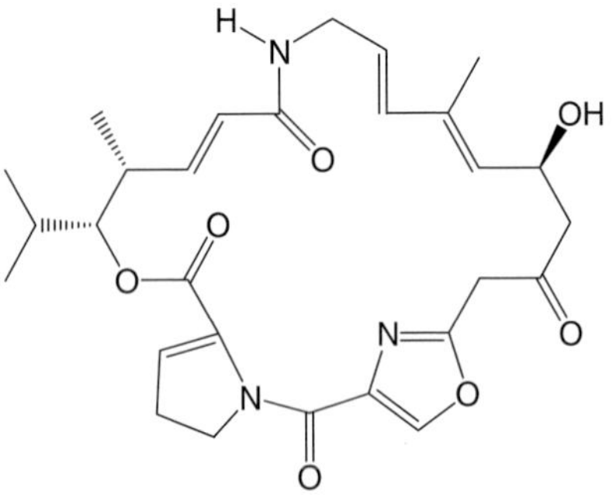

Like the other streptogramin, pristinamycin, virginiamycin is made of two subunits, virginiamycin S1 and virginiamycin M1. Dermatitis was quite common in people using the formerly available topical virginiamycin. Occupational dermatitis was observed in the pharmaceutical industry, in breeders, and in a surgeon who used topical virginiamycin on postoperative wounds (personal observation).

Suggested Reading

Rudzki E, Rebandel P (1984) Contact sensitivity to antibiotics. Contact Dermatitis 11:41–42

Tennstedt D, Dumont-Fruytier M, Lachapelle JM (1978) Occupational allergic contact dermatitis to virginiamycin, an antibiotic used as a food additive for pigs and poultry. Contact Dermatitis 4:133–134

409. Zinc bis-Dibutyldithiocarbamate

Zinc *N,N*-Dibutyldithiocarbamate

CAS Registry Number [136–23–2]

A rubber chemical, used as a vulcanization accelerator. It can also be contained in paints, glue removers, and anticorrosive. It was contained in "carba-mix."

Suggested Reading

Condé-Salazar L, Del-Rio E, Guimaraens D, Gonzalez Domingo A (1993) Type IV allergy to rubber additives: a 10-year study of 686 cases. J Am Acad Dermatol 29:176–180

Condé-Salazar L, Guimaraens D, Villegas C, Romero A, Gonzalez MA (1995) Occupational allergic contact dermatitis in construction workers. Contact Dermatitis 35:226–230

Kiec-Swierczynska M (19959 Occupational sensitivity to rubber. Contact Dermatitis 32:171–172

410. Zinc *bis*-Diethyldithiocarbamate

Zinc *N,N*-Diethyldithiocarbamate, Diethyldithiocarbamic Acid Zinc Salt

CAS Registry Number [14324–55–1]

Diethyldithiocarbamate zinc is a rubber component used as a vulcanization accelerator. It can be responsible for rubber dermatitis in health personnel. It was contained in "carba-mix."

Suggested Reading

Condé-Salazar L, Del-Rio E, Guimaraens D, Gonzalez Domingo A (1993) Type IV allergy to rubber additives: a 10-year study of 686 cases. J Am Acad Dermatol 29:176–180

Kiec-Swierczynska M (1995) Occupational sensitivity to rubber. Contact Dermatitis 32:171–172

Vaneckova J, Ettler K (1994) Hypersensitivity to rubber surgical gloves in healthcare personnel. Contact Dermatitis 31:266–267

Von Hintzenstern J, Heese A, Koch HU, Peters KP, Hornstein OP (1991) Frequency, spectrum and occupational relevance of type IV allergies to rubber chemicals. Contact Dermatitis 24:244–252

411. Zinc bis-Dimethyldithiocarbamate

Ziram

CAS Registry Number [137–30–4]

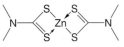

Ziram is a rubber vulcanization accelerator, of the dithiocarbamate group. Sensitization was reported in several patients. Ziram is also used as a fungicide and can cause contact dermatitis in agricultural workers.

Suggested Reading

Kiec-Swierczynska M (1995) Occupational sensitivity to rubber. Contact Dermatitis 32:171–172

Manuzzi P, Borrello P, Misciali C, Guerra L (1988) Contact dermatitis due to Ziram and Maneb. Contact Dermatitis 19:148

412. Zinc Ethylene-bis-Dithiocarbamate

Zineb, Zinc *N,N'*-Ethylenebisdithiocarbamate

CAS Registry Number [12122–67–7]

Zineb is a pesticide of the dithiocarbamate group. Sensitization can occur in gardeners and florists.

Suggested Reading

Crippa M, Misquith L, Lonati A, Pasolini G (1990) Dyshidrotic eczema and sensitization to dithiocarbamates in a florist. Contact Dermatitis 23: 203–204

Jung HD, Honemann W, Kloth C, Lubbe D, Pambor M, Quednow C, Ratz KH, Rothe A, Tarnick M (1989) Kontaktekzem durch Pestizide in der Deutschen Demokratischen Republik. Dermatol Monatsschr 175: 203–214

O'Malley M, Rodriguez P, Maibach HI (1995) Pesticide patch testing: California nursery workers and controls. Contact Dermatitis 32:61–62

413. Zinc Propylene-bis-Dithiocarbamate

Propineb, Zinc *N,N'*-Propylene-1,2-bis-Dithiocarbamate

CAS Registry Number [12071–83–9]

Propineb is a dithiocarbamate compound, which is used as a fungicide. Sensitization was reported in agricultural workers.

Suggested Reading

Jung HD, Honemann W, Kloth C, Lubbe D, Pambor M, Quednow C, Ratz KH, Rothe A, Tarnick M (1989) Kontaktekzem durch Pestizide in der Deutschen Demokratischen Republik. Dermatol Monatsschr 175: 203–214

Nishioka K, Takahata H (2000) Contact allergy due to propineb. Contact Dermatitis 43:310

Patch Testing with the Patients' Own Products

PETER J. FROSCH, JOHANNES GEIER, WOLFGANG UTER, AN GOOSSENS

Commercially available patch test kits (standard series and various supplementary series) are the basis of a diagnostic work-up if an allergic contact dermatitis is to be confirmed. However, various investigators have shown that this way of testing is not sufficient. Menné et al. [20] found in a multicenter study that the European Standard Series detects only 37–73% of the responsible allergens in patients with contact dermatitis. The additional and/or separately tested allergens were positive in 5–23%; the authors emphasize the necessity of testing with the products actually used by the patient. In Italy, an analysis of 230 patients referred to a contact clinic because of suspected occupational contact dermatitis showed that the standard series alone detected 69.9% of all cases considered to be of an allergic nature [22]; 26.3% of all allergic cases were positive only to supplementary series. The agents most commonly responsible for allergic contact dermatitis were metals and *para*-phenylenediamine.

In a German study of the IVDK network, the data of 2,460 patients tested between 1989 and 1992 were evaluated [5]. In 208 patients (8.5%) type IV sensitizations were found to a total of 289 materials. In 44% of these cases only the patients' own products were patch test positive and thought to be clinically relevant.

In a subsequent analysis of 1998–2002 data, 8.6% of 3,621 patients had a positive patch test reaction to their own skin-care products additionally patch tested. Of 1,333 patients, 5.3% were tested positive to their own bath and shower products. In about one-third of the patients reacting to either product category, further positive tests to commercial allergens were not observed [1, 29].

The materials most frequently tested are usually topical medications, cosmetics of various types, rubber and leather products.

The group of Kanerva has published an impressive series of papers in which patch testing with the patients' own industrial chemicals has provided the main clue as to the causative agent of allergic contact dermatitis [16]. Various constituents of plastic materials, epoxy glues and paints, reactive dyes, and industrial enzymes were identified after chemical analysis. With regard to isocyanates present in polyurethane resins, for example, it was found that among 22 occupationally related cases, 21 reacted to the isocyanates obtained from the companies involved (13×) or to diaminodiphenylmethane (marker for isocyanate allergy), but only 1 reacted to the commercially available isocyanate, diphenylmethane diisocyanate or MDI (Trolab, Chemotechnique) [11]. Indeed, Frick et al. [7], when analyzing 14 commercial preparations of MDI, found that in most cases its concentration did not match the one stated on the label. Moreover, the isocyanates tested are not always representative of the mixtures used in industry.

Recently, reports were published on contact allergy to the patients' perfume where the current fragrance mix and the commercially available major allergens of perfume remained negative. After repeated testing with various fractions of perfumes the causative allergens were identified: Lilial [9] and coumarin [21]. The experience with perfumes has shown that in this dynamic field, with rapid changes in trendy attractive smells, the consumer is exposed to a wide array of chemicals that may cause sensitization. This subject is reviewed in detail in Chap.31, Sect. 31.1. Further examples documenting the high value of testing with the patients' own products are published elsewhere [17–19, 28]. In this field and in many industrial areas, patch testing with merely the standard and supplementary series will always be inadequate until new allergens have been identified, their clinical relevance has been confirmed by several study groups, and they are eventually included in a test series.

In the following we want to give guidelines for testing with patients' own materials in order to harmonize this approach in daily practice. Knowledge in this field is often minimal and profound mistakes are made. For example, concentrated biocides or plastic monomers are applied under occlusion in undiluted form causing bullous or ulcerative lesions and possibly active sensitization. In contrast, the material is not infrequently diluted too much or in an inappropriate vehicle resulting in a false-negative reaction.

The guidelines are presented mainly in tables in order to be used at the work bench by technicians. They contain essential information; for more detailed information the reader is referred to other chapters in this book (particularly Chap. 49) and the pertinent references listed at the end.

1.1 Information on the Test Material Before Patch Testing

Never apply coded material obtained from a manufacturer without knowing details about the chemical regarding its toxicity and appropriate test concentration. Major cosmetic manufacturers now have a safety department that will supply this information and often provide the ingredients at adequate dilutions and a vehicle for patch testing. However, some tend to supply the ingredients in dilutions as used in the products, producing false-negative reactions on patch testing. Unfortunately, this cooperative attitude is rare with manufacturers of industrial products (e.g., metalworking fluids, glues, paints, etc.). The material safety data sheets provide only basic information and do not list all allergologically relevant ingredients. In addition, the producer selling the product is often unaware of contaminants or materials under a different nomenclature (i.e., the manufacturer denies the presence of colophony but admits that abietic acid, the major allergen of colophony, is present in a cooling fluid). In a recent study from Finland on dental restorative materials, a high discrepancy was found between the listing of acrylates/methacrylates in material safety data sheets and the presence of these materials as detected by chemical analytical methods. 2-Hydroxyethyl methacrylate (2-HEMA), bisphenol A glycidyl methacrylate (bis-GMA), ethyleneglycol dimethacrylate (EGDMA), triethylene glycol dimethacrylate (TREGDMA), and (di)urethane dimethacrylate were either omitted completely as ingredients or not listed as often as appropriate. The authors analyzed glues, composite resins, and glass isomers [13].

The German network IVDK has established a model project [27] supporting the breakdown testing of cosmetic products. In cooperation with the manufacturers, the inquiring dermatologist will receive a recommendation on how to test the product ingredients, and which constituents not present in the standard or additional series might be a potential allergen. These are then provided in a test kit supplied by the manufacturer (this service is limited to Germany). Ideally, the test results are fed back to the data center, and are added to the database for the identification of putative "new" allergens – a system similar to the "cosmetovigilance" established in France [30].

1.1.1 Test Method

1.1.1.1 Skin Tests

Methodological details regarding dilution, vehicle, pH measurement, open test, closed patch test, repetitive open application test (ROAT), and use test are dealt with in Chap. 22. In Dortmund we found large Finn chambers (12 mm diameter) useful for testing cosmetics with low irritancy (e.g., moisturizers, lip cosmetics, sunscreens, eye drops [14]; Fig. 1).

The semi-open test as described by Dooms-Goossens [6] is particularly helpful if strong irritancy under occlusion is suspected, e.g., in the case of shampoos, liquid soaps, nail varnish, and also industrial products such as glues, paints, inks, varnishes, etc. The golden rule is that when a subject comes into direct skin contact with such a product (either on purpose, e.g., cleaning products, or accidentally, e.g., soluble oils, paints), then the product may be tested in this way. Corrosive or other toxic materials (pH <3 or >10) that are normally used in closed systems only or with protection from appropriate clothing are excluded from testing. The material is applied to the skin with a cotton swab (about 15 µl) on a small area (2×2 cm), left to dry (possibly dabbing with another Q-tip or tissue), and is then covered with acrylic tape (e.g., Micropore, 3M) (Fig. 2).

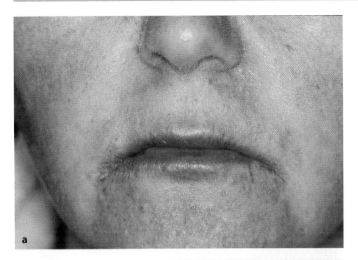

Fig. 1a, b.
Severe cheilitis with eczema-
tous pruritic lesions in the
perioral region after long-
term use of a lipstick for dry
lips (**a**). The patch test with
the lipstick "as is" in a large
Finn chamber showed a
weak doubtful reaction (**b**).
Breakdown testing with the
ingredients provided by the
manufacturer revealed a
contact allergy to dexpan-
thenol. The dermatitis
cleared rapidly after discon-
tinuance of the lipstick

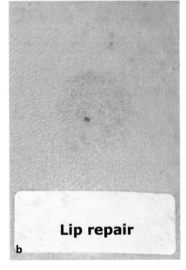

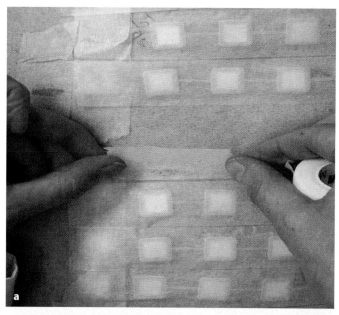

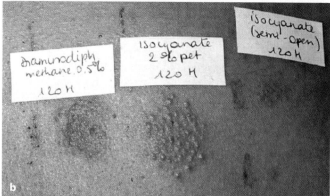

Fig. 2a, b. Semi-open test: after applying the test material with a cotton swab, the completely dried area is covered with acrylic tape (a). Comparison of positive reactions obtained with a semi-open test to the patient's own isocyanate solution and a patch test with its dilution at 2% in petrolatum (b); there was also a positive reaction to diaminodiphenylmethane as a marker for isocyanate contact allergy

1.1.1.2 pH

At pH 4–9, very few irritant reactions are caused by the acidity or alkalinity itself [3]. The buffering solutions listed in Table 1 can be used to dilute water-soluble materials.

1.1.1.3 Dilution

Solid materials can be tested "as is," placing scrapings or cut pieces in the test chamber, or they can be applied on acrylic tape thus avoiding pressure effects. In this way, positive reactions may be obtained to small pieces of glove, shoes, rubber, or to scrapings of (hard) plastic materials (Fig. 3). However, the reactions often turn out to be false negative because the concentration of the sensitizer is too low or the sensitizer is not released. Alternatively, pressure or friction effects of sharp particles may cause some sort of irritant reaction, which should, however, be clearly identifiable as such. Depending on the material, the sensitizer can be extracted with water or solvents (Table 2; [16]).

The correct dilution of materials for patch testing often presents a technical problem because the calculation basis is not clear to every technician. Therefore Table 3 provides a practical guideline

Table 1. Composition of acid buffer solution, pH 4.7, and alkaline buffer solution, pH 9.9 [3]

Compound	Concentration	% of total volume
Acid buffer, pH 4.7		
Sodium acetate	0.1 N (8.2 g CH_3COONa/l aqua)	50
Acetic acid	0.1 N (6.0 g CH_3COOH/l aqua)	50
Alkaline buffer, pH 9.9		
Sodium carbonate	0.1 M (10.6 g Na_2CO_3/l aqua)	50
Sodium bicarbonate	0.1 M (8.4 g $NaHCO_3/l$ aqua)	50

Fig. 3a–c.
Contact dermatitis of the ear
due to a hearing aid (**a, b**).
Patch testing with fine scrapings of the plastic material
was strongly positive (**c**). In
subsequent testing with the
plastic series the patient also
showed a positive reaction to
2-hydroxyethyl methacrylate
(*2-HEMA*) which was a
component of the hearing
aid as the manufacturer
confirmed

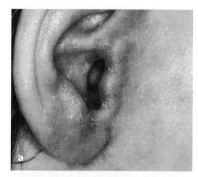

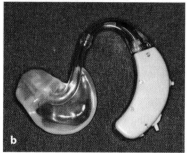

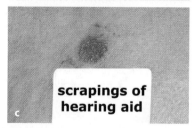

scrapings of
hearing aid

Table 2. Materials suitable for extraction and recommended solvents [16]

Material	Solvent
Paper	Ethanol
Plants and wood dusts	Acetone, ether, ethanol or water
Plastics, e.g., gloves	Acetone
Rubber, e.g., gloves	Acetone or water
Textiles	Ethanol

Table 3. Recipe for diluting materials for patch testing [24]

Desired percentage dilution (%)	Quantity (µl) to be mixed in 10 ml of vehicle
0.1	10
0.5	50
1.0	100
2.0	200
5.0	500 (0.5 ml)
10	1000 (1.0 ml)

for diluting liquid materials. For solid materials the dilution is performed based on a weight:volume basis.

1.1.2 Control Tests

When a reaction to a new material is observed which suggests a contact allergy based on morphology and development over time, control tests on human volunteers should be performed. This procedure is, however, now a great problem in some countries. In most German University departments, for instance, the approval of the ethics committee has to be obtained beforehand and each volunteer has to provide informed consent.

2.1 Product Categories for Patch Testing

2.1.1 Decorative Cosmetics, Sunscreens, Toiletries (Tables 4 and 5)

Many allergens are included in the standard series, the series for vehicles, emulsifiers, and preservatives. Fine fragrances may contain ingredients that are not present in commercially available test compounds. Perfumes in alcoholic solutions can be tested as is – occasionally slight irritant reactions (erythema without infiltration) might occur; the frequency of these reactions can be reduced by allowing the patch to dry before applied to the skin [15].

Table 4. Testing of decorative cosmetics and sunscreens. Abbreviations for vehicles in the following tables: *ac* acetone, *MEK* methyl ethyl ketone, *oo* olive oil, *pet* petrolatum, *w* water

Cosmetic/sunscreen	Concentration	Comment
Eye make-up		
Eye liner	As is	
Eye shadow	As is	
Mascara	As is	Semi-open test first, allow to dry (solvents)
Make-up cleanser	As is	Semi-open test first, irritation possible (amphoteric or other detergents)
Facial make-up		
Rouge	As is	
Powder	As is	
Foundation	As is	
Lip stick	As is	Photopatch when sunscreens are incorporated
Moisturizers		
Creams, ointments, lotions	As is	Irritation possible; positive patch test reaction should be confirmed by ROAT or use test. Photopatch test when sunscreens present
Bleaching creams	As is	
Sunscreens	As is	Photopatch test including active ingredients as commercially available
Self-tanning creams	As is	
Perfumed products		
Fine fragrances	As is	Allow to dry. Photopatch if clinical findings suggest actinic dermatitis
Eau de Toilette	As is	
After shave	As is	
Deodorants		
Spray, roll on, stick	As is	Allow to dry. Irritation possible. Often false negative, ROAT!
Shaving products		
Cream	1% (w)	Semi-open with product as is first. Irritation possible under occlusion
Soap	1% (w)	

Table 5. Testing of cleaning products

Product type	Concentration	Comment
Soap bar	1% (w)	Irritation possible; use test
Shampoo	1% (w)	
Shower gel	1% (w)	
Bathing foam	0.1% (w)	
Toothpaste	1% (w)	

Many moisturizing creams for the face now contain sunscreens as "anti-aging factors."

The detergents that are active ingredients (sodium lauryl sulfate, lauryl ether sulfates, sulfosuccinic esters, isethionates) are not important allergens. They cause irritant reactions at dilutions at 1–0.5% in most subjects, particularly in patients with sensitive skin. Perfumes and preservatives may be relevant allergens in this category of products [1, 29]). Cocamidopropyl betaine has caused allergic patch test reactions for some time. Now the major allergen (3-dimethylaminopropylamine) has been identified and removed from this major detergent in shampoos and shower gels.

2.2.2 Hairdressing, Depilatory, and Nail Cosmetics (Table 6)

Major allergens are listed in the standard and supplementary series. However, as the group of Menné has recently shown, not all cases of contact dermatitis from hair dyes are identified by *para*-phenylenediamine (PPD) and derivatives [25]. Therefore individual testing with the patients' own hair dyes might be necessary. To reduce the risk of active sensitization an open test must precede the closed patch test. Recently, an epidemic of allergic contact dermatitis from epilating products in France and Belgium has been elucidated [10]. By testing with the commercial products and the ingredients, it was found that modified colophonium derivatives were the main allergens (although in most patients the colophonium of the standard series was negative); further allergens were methoxy

Table 6. Testing of hair dressing products and nail cosmetics

Product	Concentration	Comment
Hair dyes	2% (w)	Active sensitization possible! Semi-open test: 5 drops dye and 5 drops oxidizing agent. If negative after 48 h, closed patch test with 2%
Hair spray	As is	Allow to dry. Irritation possible
Hair gel	As is	Semi-open test first
Depilatory	As is	Semi-open test first. Irritation possible (do not occlude)
Nail lacquer	As is	Always semi-open test only
Nail lacquer remover		Do not test (highly irritating)
Glues for artificial nails	1% and 0.1% (MEK)	Semi-open test as is. Most glues are cured with UV light

PEG-22/dodecyl glycol copolymer and lauryl alcohol, present in the accompanying skin conditioning tissue.

2.2.3 Topical Medicaments

Most topical medicaments used for dermatological conditions can be tested undiluted. Few contain irritating constituents (benzoyl peroxide, tretinoin, mustard, capsaicin, liquid antiseptic agents such as those containing PVP-iodine and nonoxynol, or quaternary ammonium, etc.) – these must be tested in a dilution series. Chapter 35 on topical drugs lists many chemicals as active ingredients that have been identified as contact allergens by patch testing the material of the patient.

2.2.4 Medical Applicances

EKG contact gel	As is
Various aids from plastic materials (prosthesis, hearing aid)	Scrapings, undiluted
Implantations, materials for osteosynthesis	
Metals in standard series	
Methylmethacrylate	2% pet
Palacos® and monomer liquids	Do not test undiluted

Do not test parts of osteosynthesis materials with sharp edges (irritant reactions)

Most patients with a metal allergy (nickel, chromium, cobalt) tolerate implanted metals. Sensitization by implanted materials after a variable latent period of weeks or months, however, has been reported; overall it seems to be rare with modern metal alloys. Predictive testing is not indicated.

2.2.5 Dental Prosthesis and Other Dental Restorative Materials

Fine scrapings of the prosthesis can be tested with a large Finn chamber, physiological saline added. An allergic contact stomatitis caused by these materials is extremely rare. Sensitizations by acrylates may occur, although these are primarily seen in dental technicians on the hands, by daily contacts at work.

2.2.6 Disinfecting Agents

These materials are often irritating under occlusion for 48 h in a patch test. Therefore, a semi-open test should always be performed first (Table 7). Furthermore, it might be necessary to test with the

Table 7. Testing of disinfecting agents

Product	Concentration	Comment
Hand disinfection	As is	Semi-open test first. Closed patch test may be irritating. Use test. Test ingredients!
Disinfecting agents for instruments, floors, etc.	1%, 0.1%, 0.01%	Semi-open test first. Often contain strong irritants

individual constituents of the product to detect a contact allergy (e.g., to hand disinfecting agents).

2.2.7 Clothing

A piece of the suspected material – textiles, gloves, shoes – (2 × 2 cm moistened with saline solution) is applied under occlusion for 48 h on the back.

Textile dyes, formaldehyde resins, and thioureas can be identified by further testing with the supplementary series. Acid dyes may actively sensitize if tested at high concentrations. Therefore, new dyes brought in by the patient must be initially tested at high dilution. In this context, patch testing with thin-layer chromatograms can serve as an elegant adjunct to quickly identify contact allergy to a certain ingredient of a mixture, such as a textile dye, although the (variable, possibly high) detection limit may yield false-negative results [4].

2.2.8 Pesticides

Most reactions to pesticides are irritant and pose the hazard of systemic toxicity by percutaneous absorption. Therefore, we do not recommend patch testing with pesticides unless there is strong evidence for allergic contact dermatitis. Detailed information about toxicity must be obtained before sequential testing (open test, semi-open test, closed patch test).

2.2.9 Detergents for Household Cleaning

General recommendation: 1% and 0.1% (water), semi-open test first, control for pH!

It is usually the additives, such as perfumes, preservatives, dyes etc., that are the sensitizers, rather than the detergents, although the frequency of contact allergy to this type of product is apparently often overestimated [2].

Harsh detergents contain quaternary ammonium compounds, which are highly irritating.

2.2.10 Food Stuff

In food handlers and bakers a protein contact dermatitis must be excluded by prick and scratch chamber testing.

2.2.10.1 Scratch Chamber Testing [23]

After four scarifications with a fine needle, the test material is applied under a large Finn chamber for 24 h. Readings are taken after 24 and 48 h. With fruits and vegetables, irritant reactions are quite frequent.

For bakers, the flours used, the spices, and enzymes must be tested in prick and scratch chamber tests (amylase 1% in water).

In rare cases an exposure test with the dough squeezed in the hands for 20 min might confirm a suspected protein contact dermatitis.

2.2.11 Plants

Patch testing with pieces of plants is not recommended in general because irritant reactions are frequent and active sensitization may occur, although direct application on acrylic tape and not occluded by a chamber is less apt to do so. The commercially available and standardized materials for patch testing (sesquiterpene lactone mix, primin, Compositae mix, diallyl sulfide, tulipaline, etc.) are safe and identify most cases of plant dermatitis. In professional gardeners sensitization to various plants might occur.

In cases of recalcitrant plant dermatitis and unproductive patch testing with commercially available allergens, it may be worthwhile producing an extract of the suspected plant according to Hausen [12]. The pertinent features are listed in Table 8.

Plant extracts may be highly irritating. Therefore, adequate control tests must be performed in every case. It is self evident that the exact botanical classification is necessary before starting any investigative work.

2.12 Woods

Fine wood dust moistened with physiological saline can be patch tested with a Finn chamber or on adhesive acrylic tape. Exotic woods can be strongly irritating and sensitizing (teak, rosewood, Macoré) – these should be diluted to at least 10% in petrolatum (sensitization might occur even at lower concentrations in rare cases).

Turpentine and colophony (peroxides) are the major allergens of conifers (pine, spruce, larch).

Table 8. The production of a plant extract for patch testing according to Hausen [12]

1. Obtaining a concentrate of the plant juice by cutting, pressing or smashing in a mortar; dilution with water by 1:10 and 1:100

2. Short extraction with diethylether (60–90 s). Working with ether is dangerous because of its explosive nature. If there is no suitable laboratory equipment available (rotation evaporation under an exhaust system), a practical alternative is the use of large open glassware filled with the solvent and the plant, left open in the air for about 1 h

3. Tulips, lilies, alstroemeria and other Liliaceae are extracted more efficiently with ethanol

4. After evaporation of the solvent the extract is incorporated into a suitable vehicle: water, ethanol, methanol, acetone, acidic acid ester, methylethylketone or plant oil. The use of petrolatum is also possible. Dilution series to start with: 1:10, 1:100, 1:1000. The material should be kept in a refrigerator

2.13 Office Work

Reactions to paper and cardboard are usually irritant in nature, particularly in atopics. In rare cases sensitizations to colophony or formaldehyde resins may be relevant. A piece of paper (2×2 cm, moistened with physiological saline) is applied occlusively for 2 days. NCR (carbonless) paper can be tested in the same way after rubbing it firmly to release the encapsulated dye. Diethylendiamine and colophony have been identified as allergens in NCR paper [17]. Telefax paper may also contain contact allergens (colophony, Bisphenol A). According to Karlberg and Lidén [31] testing with paper extracts (in acetone or methanol) is more reliable than a patch test with the paper as is.

Other materials that may be relevant to chronic hand eczema in office workers are:

- Rubber articles
- Glues (colophony, various resins)
- Woods (desk tops, handles)
- Metals (nickel in metallic objects such as perforators, pens, etc.)
- Plants
- Liquid soaps, hand creams used at the work place

2.14 Construction Materials

- Concrete
- Cement
- Resins for various purposes
- Tile setting materials

Testing with the material as is under occlusion is absolutely contra-indicated because of high irritancy. A semi-open test might be indicated in cases with a high suspicion of contact allergy, particularly when resins are involved and testing with the standard and supplementary series remains negative. The main allergen in cement is potassium dichromate, which is present in the standard series. Fast-curing cements contain epoxy resins, which are increasingly recognized as major allergens in the construction industry but also in other industrial areas (painting, metal, electronics, and plastic). The epoxy resin of the standard series is insufficient to detect all cases of relevant epoxy resin allergies, as has been shown by a large German multicenter study [8]. Sometimes acrylic resins may also be present.

2.2.15 Paints, Lacquers

The chemical composition of paints and lacquers is very complex. Acrylates of various types are added for rapid curing. In the so-called biologic paints turpentine and colophony are often present. Isothiazolinones are frequently used in water-based wall paints. Before patch testing is performed with these products detailed information from the manufacturer should be obtained. Semi-open tests can be performed. As a guideline the concentrations as listed in Table 9 can be used.

2.2.16 Greases and Oils

These materials primarily used for lubrication rarely produce an allergic contact dermatitis. They are not very irritating except for hydraulic oils. Table 10 provides the recommended test concentrations.

2.2.17 Metalworking Fluids (MWF)

Metalworking fluids are indispensable for the processing of metal parts. Their chemical composition varies with the purpose and type of metal. Material safety data sheets usually do not contain all relevant allergological information. The most important allergens are rust preventives/emulsifiers, resin acids from distilled tall oil, and biocides. Table 11 provides guidelines for testing with MWF [26].

Table 9. Testing of paints, lacquers and solvents. Semi-open test first for all paints or lacquers

Product	Concentration	Comment
One component (water based, e.g., wall paints)	10–100% (w)	
One component (solvent or oil-based, e.g., paints for wood, iron, etc.)	1–10% (pet)	
Diisocyanate hardeners of polyurethane paints or lacquers	2–5% (pet)	
Paints containing epoxy,	0.1–1.0% (pet)	Obtain detailed polyesters or acrylics information on chemical composition first. Test conc. may be raised to 10% for some paints (see Chap. 34 on plastics)
Organic solvents		
Aliphatic, cycloaliphatic	1–10% (pet)	
Aromatic	1–5% (pet)	
Chlorinated	0.1–1% (pet)	
Esters	1–10% (pet)	

Table 10. Testing of technical greases and oils

Product	Concentration	Comment
Lubricating grease	As is and 20% (pet)	Semi-open test first
Lubricating oils	As is, 50%, 10% (oo)	
Hydraulic oils	1% (oo)	

Table 11. Testing of metalworking fluids (*MWF*) – for details see Chap. 33

Product	Concentration (%)	Comment
Water-based	5 (w)	The usual workplace concentration of fresh MWF is 4–8%. Test a freshly diluted MWF at 5%, the used one as is (provided the concentration at the workplace is less than 8% – otherwise use a dilution of at least 1:1)
Oil-based	50 (oo)	

The most common mistake when testing water-based MWF is that the concentrate brought in by the patient is patch tested without further dilution. This usually produces severe irritant, sometimes ulcerative, lesions. The concentrate is usually diluted to 4–8% by adding water in the circulatory system of the machine. Metal workers often come into contact with this dilution of the MWF and develop a chronic irritant contact dermatitis (Fig. 4).

Perfumes as "odor masks" are often added and may produce an allergic contact dermatitis. The same holds true for isothiazolinones and other biocides, which are also often added as "system cleaners" in excessive concentrations during the use cycle of a MWF in order to prevent degradation and bad odors. Therefore, testing of both the fresh and the used MWF is obligatory.

2.2.18 Rubber Chemicals

Rubber products can be patch tested as is. This may be particularly worthwhile with protective gloves, rubber masks or other materials with prolonged direct skin contact. Often the usual rubber ingredients available for patch testing remain negative. The isolation of the allergen in rubber products is extremely difficult due to the complex chemical nature and the numerous additives used for maintaining the desired technical features. As a guideline, accelerators, anti-oxidants, and other materials provided by a cooperative

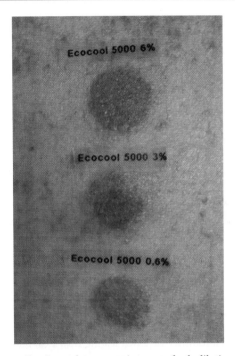

Fig. 4. Strong allergic patch test reactions to a fresh dilution series of a metalworking fluid brought in by a patient with chronic occupational hand eczema (use concentration at the work place was 6% in water). He also showed positive reactions to colophony (2+), abietic acid (3+), monoethanolamine (1+), and 2-(2-aminoethoxy)ethanol (diglycolamine) (1+). These materials are often present in metalworking fluids and may cause relevant sensitizations

manufacturer can be tested at 1% in petrolatum. Positive reactions require further dilutions and testing on control persons.

2.2.19 Glues and Adhesives

This group of products is nowadays ubiquitous and frequently used at home for production and repairs in various areas. Glues are often irritating in undiluted form. Testing with acrylates in inadequate dilutions can cause active sensitization. The test concentrations as listed in Table 12 provide a guideline only; before patch testing an unknown new material, detailed information from the manufacturer should be obtained. Testing should always start with a semi-open test to avoid strong irritant reactions or active sensitization.

2.2.20 Plastic Materials

Testing with this group of chemicals is recommended with the commercially available substances for patch testing of major manufacturers. These materials have been validated on large groups of patients and the patch test concentrations can be considered as safe and nonsensitizing.

Most patients have contact only with the end product after complete curing and containing no monomers as irritating or sensitizing components. However, as described in detail in Chap. 34 on plastic materials exceptions to this rule do occur and relevant sensitization may only be detected by patch testing fine dust particles of the plastic product or with all ingredients after time-consuming dilution series. Patch testing with a thin-layer chromatogram of a resin of unknown composition may be an interesting option to screen for the causative agent [4].

Table 12. Testing of glues and adhesives

Product	Concentration	Comment
Adhesive tapes	As is	
Glues (excluding epoxy, formaldehyde resin and acrylic)		Semi-open test first. Allow to dry when patch testing
Dispersion glues	10–100% (pet or w)	
Solvent-based contact glues	1–10% (pet)	
Cyanoacrylate	2% (pet)	Strong irritant, rare allergen. Semi-open test first

A few of these materials are carcinogenic and may cause bronchial asthma (for example the group of isocyanates). Therefore, these materials must be handled with great caution.

2.2.21 Do Not Test

In general, the following materials should not be tested because they are known as strong irritants but not as contact allergens (with few exceptions).

Patch testing may be performed only if there is high suspicion of contact allergy by history and clinical findings. Then an open and semi-open test should precede closed patch testing (dilution series from 0.1% to 1%).

- Astringents (e.g., $AgNO_3$)
- Anti freeze
- Car wax
- Gasoline
- Diesel
- Floor wax
- Lime
- Organic solvents (various types)
- Kerosene
- Metal chips (coarse)
- Rust remover
- White spirit
- Toluene
- Toilet cleaners and other strong caustic cleaning agents
- Cement, concrete

All products that have a strong pungent odor and/or contain organic solvents should be tested for pH (see above). If an open and semi-open test is negative a dilution series starting with a very high dilution can be performed under occlusion (maximum 24 h, locating on the medial aspect of the upper arm, which enables removal by the patient in case pain occurs).

If there is doubt about the nature of the patch test reaction – irritant or allergic – an expert in the field should be consulted before further testing is performed. Active sensitization of volunteers or ulcerative lesions with scar formation may be the risk of further investigative procedures.

References

1. Balzer C, Schnuch A, Geier J, Uter W (2005) Ergebnisse der Epikutantestung mit patienteneigenen Kosmetika und Körperpflegemittel im IVDK, 1998–2002. Dermatol Beruf Umwelt53:8–24

2. Belsito DV, Fransway AF, Fowler JF Jr, Sherertz EF, Maibach HI, Mark JG Jr, Mathias CG, Rietschel RL, Storrs FJ, Nethercott JR (2002) Allergic contact dermatitis to detergents: a multicenter study to assess prevalence. J Am Acad Dermatol 46(2):200–2006

3. Bruze M (1984) Use of buffer solutions for patch testing. Contact Dermatitis 10:267–269

4. Bruze M, Frick M, Persson L (2003) Patch testing with thin-layer chromatograms. Contact Dermatitis 48:278–279

5. Daecke CM (1994) Der Stellenwert patienteneigener Testsubstanzen bei der Epikutantestung. Hautarzt 45:292–298

6. Dooms-Goossens A (1995) Patch testing without a kit. In: Guin JD (ed) Practical contact dermatitis. A handbook for the practitioner. McGraw-Hill, Philadelphia, Pa., pp 63–74

7. Frick M, Zimerson E, Karlsson D et al (2004) Poor correlation between stated and found concentration of diphenylmethane-4,4´-diisocyanate (4,4´-MDI) in petrolatum patch-test preparations. Contact Dermatitis 51:73–78

8. Geier J, Lessmann H, Hillen U, Jappe U, Dickel H, Koch P et al (2004) An attemt to improve diagnostics of contact allergy due to epoxy resin systems. First results of the multicentre study EPOX 2002. Contact Dermatitis 51:263–272

9. Giménez Arnau E, Andersen KE, Bruze M, Frosch PJ, Johansen JD, Menné T, Rastogie SE, White IR, Lepoittevin JP (2000) Identification of Lilial® as a fragrance sensitizer in a perfume by bioassay-guided chemical fractionation and structure-activity relationships. Contact Dermatitis 43:351–358

10. Goossens A, Armingaud P, Avenel-Audran M et al (2002) An epidemic of allergic contact dermatitis due to epilating products. Contact Dermatitis 46:67–70

11. Goossens A, Detienne T, Bruze M (2002) Occupational allergic contact dermatitis caused by isocyanates. Contact Dermatitis 47:304–308

12. Hausen BM (1988) Allergiepflanzen, Pflanzengifte. Handbuch und Atlas der allergieinduzierenden Wild- und Kulturpflanzen. 1988 Ecomed Verlag, Landsberg Lech

13. Henriks-Eckerman M, Suuronen K, Jolanki R, Alanko K (2004) Methacrylates in dental restorative materials. Contact Dermatitis 50:233–237
14. Herbst RA, Uter W, Pirker C, Geier J, Frosch PJ (2004) Allergic and nonallergic periorbital dermatitis: patch test results of the Information Network of the Departments of Dermatology during a 5-year period. Contact Dermatitis 51:13–19
15. Johansen JD, Frosch PJ, Rastogi SC, Menné T (2001) Testing with fine fragrances in eczema patients. Contact Dermatitis 44:304–307
16. Jolanki R, Estlander T, Alanko K, Kanerva L (2000) Patch testing with a patient's own materials handled at work. In: Kanerva L, Elsner P, Wahlberg JE, Maibach HI (eds) Handbook of occupational dermatology.Springer-Verlag, Berlin Heidelberg New York, pp 375–383
17. Lange-Ionescu S, Bruze M, Gruvberger B, Zimerson E, Frosch PJ (2000) Kontaktallergie durch kohlefreies Durchschlagpapier. Dermat Beruf Umwelt 48:183–187
18. Magerl A, Heiss R, Frosch PJ (2001) Allergic contact dermatitis from zinc ricinoleate in a deodorant and glyceryl ricinoleate in a lipstick. Contact Dermatitis 44:119–121
19. Magerl A, Pirker C, Frosch PJ (2003) Allergisches Kontaktekzem durch Schellack und 1,3-Butylenglykol in einem Eyliner. Journal Deutsch Dermatolog Gesellsch 1:300–302
20. Menné T, Dooms-Goossens A, Wahlberg JE, White IR, Shaw S (1992) How large a proportion of contact sensitivities are diagnosed with the European standard series? Contact Dermatitis 26:201–202
21. Mutterer V, Giménez Arnau E, Lepoittevin JP, Johansen JD, Frosch PJ, Menné T, Andersen KE, Bruze M, Rastogi SC, White IR (1999) Identification of coumarin as the sensitizer in a patient sensitive to her own perfume but negative to the fragrance mix. Contact Dermatitis 40:196–199
22. Nettis E, Marcandrea M, Colonardi MC, Paradiso MT, Ferrannini, Tursi A (2003) Results of standard series patch testing in patients with occupational allergic contact dermatitis. Allergy 58:1304–1307
23. Niinimäki A (1987) Scratch-chamber tests in food handler dermatitis. Contact Dermatitis 16:11–20
24. Sherertz EF, Byers SV (1997) Estimating dilutions for patch testing skin care products: a practical method. Am J Contact Derm 8:181–182
25. Sosted H, Basketter DA, Estrada E, Johansen JD, Patlewicz GY (2004) Ranking of hair dye substances according to predicted sensitization potency: quantitative structure-activity relationships. Contact Dermatitis 51:241–254
26. Tiedemann KH, Zöllner G, Adam M et al (2002) Empfehlungen für die Epikutantestung bei Verdacht auf Kontaktallergie durch Kühlschmierstoffe. 2. Hinweise zur Arbeitsstofftestung. Dermatol Beruf Umwelt 50:180–189
27. Uter W, Geier J, Lessmann H, Schnuch A (1999) Unverträglichkeitsreaktionen gegen Körperpflege- und Haushaltsprodukte: Was ist zu tun? Die Informations- und Dokumentationsstelle für Kontaktallergien (IDOK) des Informationsverbundes Dermatologischer Kliniken (IVDK). Deutsche Dermatologe 47:211–214

28. Uter W, Balzer C, Geier J, Schnuch A, Frosch PJ (2005) Ergebnisse der Epikutantestung mit patienteneigenen Parfüms, Deos und Rasierwässern. Ergebnisse des IVDK 1998–2002. Dermatol Beruf Umwelt 53: 25–36

29. Uter W, Balzer C, Geier J, Frosch PJ, Schnuch A (2005) Patch testing with patients' own cosmetics and toiletries – results of the IVDK, 1998–2002. Contact Dermatitis 53:226–233

30. Vigan M (1997) Les nouveaux allergenes des cosmetiques. La cosmetovigilance. Ann Dermatol Venereol 124:571–575

31. Karlberg AT, Lidén C (1992) Colophony (rosin) in newspapers may contribute to hand eczema. Br J Dermatol 126:161–165